Reproduction in Cattle

Third Edition

P.J.H. BALL BSc, PhD
A.R. PETERS BA, DVetMed, PhD, FRCVS, FIBiol

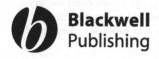

Blackwell
Publishing

Editorial Offices:
Blackwell Publishing Ltd, 9600 Garsington Road, Oxford OX4 2DQ, UK
 Tel: +44 (0)1865 776868
Blackwell Publishing Professional, 2121 State Avenue, Ames, Iowa 50014-8300, USA
 Tel: +1 515 292 0140
Blackwell Publishing Asia Pty Ltd, 550 Swanston Street, Carlton, Victoria 3053, Australia
 Tel: +61 (0)3 8359 1011

First edition published 1986 by Butterworth & Co. Publishers
Second edition published 1995 by Blackwell Science
Third edition published 2004 by Blackwell Publishing
2 2007

Library of Congress Cataloging-in-Publication Data
 Ball, P.J.H.
 Reproduction in cattle / P. Ball & A. Peters. – 3rd ed.
  p. cm.
 Rev. ed. of: Reproduction in cattle / A.R. Peters, P.J.H. Ball., 1995.
 Includes bibliographical references and index.
 ISBN 1-4051-1545-9 (pbk. : alk. paper)
 1. Cattle–Reproduction. 2. Cattle–Breeding. I. Peters, A.R. II. Peters, A.R.
Reproduction in cattle. III. Title.

 SF768.2.C3B35 2004
 636.2′08926–dc22
 2004005420

ISBN 978-1-4051-1545-2

A catalogue record for this title is available from the British Library

Set in 10 on 12.5 pt Times
by SNP Best-set Typesetter Ltd., Hong Kong

For further information on Blackwell Publishing, visit our website:
www.blackwellpublishing.com

Contents

Preface

It bears repeating from previous editions that cattle are an integral part of animal agriculture in all parts of the world. They provide the human population with products such as milk, meat, clothing, fertilizer and fuel, as well as providing draft power in many countries. Demand for some products, such as fat in meat and in milk, has declined in some markets, and in some countries (e.g., in the European Union) milk production is limited by quotas. Nevertheless, the efficient production of animal protein continues to be of vital importance. An efficient production system must maximize the output of meat and milk per unit of feed input and per animal and, in cattle production, as with other livestock systems, a high level of reproductive performance is absolutely crucial to efficient production.

Efficient reproduction results in optimum calving intervals, which in turn result in optimum production of milk and calves to be reared for beef or replacements. Furthermore, cows that fail to reproduce are culled, limiting the choice of animals available to produce replacements and thus limiting genetic progress. As awareness of the ethical issues surrounding animal production increases, this wastage becomes even more unacceptable. Welfare concerns are also increasing the pressure to avoid animal ill-health and, specifically, fertility problems. This should be regarded as a positive trend since, as will become evident in the book, improved health and welfare go hand in hand with better reproductive performance.

In the UK, the BSE epidemic and the subsequent outbreak of foot-and-mouth disease have resulted in large numbers of cattle being culled. Those that remain need to reproduce even more efficiently to provide a good choice of replacement stock. Unfortunately, however, there is evidence that dairy cattle reproductive performance in the UK and other countries where intensive dairying is practised is declining. Conception rates are now considerably lower than they were when our first edition appeared in 1986 and oestrus detection – always a major limiting factor to efficient cattle reproduction – has become considerably less effective.

In order to manage cattle reproduction and the specific problems that arise, it is important to understand the underlying physiology of the reproductive process. Thus, the third edition, as did the first two, aims to provide an integrated overview of the subject of bovine reproduction, describing the normal function of the reproductive system together with its modification by pharmacological, technological and management techniques in relation to the central theme of reproductive efficiency. The book continues to provide a general background to the field of cattle reproduction for agricultural and animal science students and as an introductory text to veterinary students and post-graduate students embarking on a career in reproductive research. Furthermore, we hope that it will be used by working veterinarians and by progressive farmers to update them on new research findings and developments in the management of cattle breeding. In this new edition we have attempted to integrate the various sections covering anatomy and physiology and those on management and animal health into a more logical sequence. We have incorporated recent findings on the physiology of the oestrous cycle and its control, as well as new techniques for monitoring and manipulating reproduction, such as oestrus synchronization, pregnancy diagnosis and embryo transfer. As before, we do not intend to provide a manual of instruction for such techniques but rather to describe and explain the principles involved. The importance of adapting management procedures to take account of changing cows and conditions is emphasized.

Reproductive efficiency, with an emphasis on the farmer's aims and requirements, is discussed in the first chapter. Most examples will be drawn from the cattle industry in the UK, with which the authors are most familiar, but the general principles can be extrapolated widely. The following chapters describe the anatomy and physiology of the male and female reproductive systems, with a detailed description of sperm production, ovarian cycles, fertilization and pregnancy. Subsequent chapters describe and discuss management procedures and techniques to maximize reproductive performance, including the vitally important detection of oestrus as well as oestrus control, artificial insemination and pregnancy diagnosis. This is followed by a description of the common infertility problems, after which a chapter on reproductive management puts these themes into a practical context. The book concludes with chapters on embryo transfer and related technologies, selection of animals for breeding and a final summary of the most important features and future trends in the control of reproduction in cattle.

We would like to record our thanks to all those people who have provided information and permission to reproduce data and illustrations, and these are acknowledged individually in the text. We are particularly grateful to Professors Hilary Dobson, Claire Wathes and Bob Webb, Drs Emma Bleach, Will Christie, Dick Esslemont, Patrick Lonergan, Tom McEvoy and Toby Mottram, and to staff of Semex, including Dr Tom Kroetsch, to staff of Cogent, including Messrs Marco Winters and Innes Drummond, and to staff of the British Society of Animal Science, including Mr Mike Steele.

P.J.H. BALL
A.R. PETERS

Chapter 1
Reproductive Efficiency in Cattle Production

In cattle production, good reproductive performance is essential to efficient management and production as a whole, although specific reproductive targets may depend to an extent on local conditions and on individual farm systems and targets. Therefore it would be helpful to give, at the outset, a brief overview of the various systems of cattle production, their requirements and the importance of reproductive efficiency in attaining them.

In some countries, especially in the tropics, much of the cattle production could be described as multi-purpose, with cows being used to provide milk, meat, clothing, fertilizer, fuel, draft power and sometimes for status or as a form of currency. However, for the most part, cattle production may be divided into two sectors: dairy production and beef production. In much of mainland Europe (excluding France) and the developing countries, the same cattle are used as a source of both beef and milk and therefore have a 'dual purpose'. The aim of breeding is to utilize individual parents of high quality in both characteristics. By contrast, in countries such as Australia, New Zealand, the USA, Canada and Israel the functions of beef and milk production have been separated and selective improvement of livestock is directed towards a single characteristic.

The situation in the UK is intermediate between these two extremes in that the beef and dairy industries are interdependent. In 1992, almost half of the animals reared for beef were dairy-bred steers, heifers and bulls. However, there is a move away from this situation as many producers recognize that the Holstein influence in breeding cow populations is undermining profitability by increasing maintenance and replacement costs and by reducing carcase grading standards of the progeny. There is thus a move towards alternative suckler replacement strategies, based on maternal beef breeds.

Dairy production

The main objective in the dairy herd is to produce milk as economically as possible. The size of enterprise varies widely. For example, in Greece most herds have below 20 cows, whereas in France most have between 10 and 40. In North America, New Zealand and Israel the majority have well in excess of 100 cows.

Table 1.1 Dairy herds with more than 100 cows as a percentage of all dairy herds (National Dairy Council, 2002).

	England and Wales	*Scotland*	*Northern Ireland*
1995	22.1	33.0	7.0
2001	32.2	43.8	14.8

Table 1.2 Recent trends in UK dairy production (National Dairy Council, 2002).

	1995	*2001*
No. of herds ('000s)	38.2	24.0
No. of cows ('000s)	2599.7	1939.1
Milk per cow (litres)	5380	6320

In the UK, the proportion of herds with more than 100 cows is increasing rapidly (Table 1.1). At the same time, the number of herds and cows has decreased markedly, whilst milk yields per cow have risen (Table 1.2). This rise is partly attributable to the increased proportion of Holstein, rather than Friesian, blood in UK dairy cows.

The main purpose of breeding is to maximize milk yield, although milk composition and other factors are becoming increasingly important. In the developed countries breeding is an advanced science, particularly where artificial insemination (AI) is practised, so that only the highest quality sires are used (see Chapter 15).

Most purebred female (heifer) calves produced are reared and kept as replacements for the milking herd. Most male calves are a by-product and are sold or reared for beef production. However, Holstein bull calves are not popular for beef suckler systems and whilst BSE export restrictions were in place, prices for bull calves were so low that they became, in effect, a worthless by-product of dairy production. A small proportion of bulls of high genetic merit might be retained as future bulls (sires). Under UK systems about the best two-thirds of cows are bred with a good quality bull, to produce purebred calves, half of which could be potential replacement heifers. A small number of very high genetic heifer calves could become the mothers of future AI stud bulls. The other third of cows tends to be crossed with a bull of a beef breed, e.g., Hereford, to produce calves with a greater potential for beef production. Such crossbred heifer calves are often utilized in beef herds as replacement suckler cows.

In intensive dairying systems, heifers are reared with the intention of calving them for the first time at two years of age. The calf is normally taken from the cow within a few days of birth and reared separately, usually receiving artificial milk substitute as a basic diet until weaning. Almost all the milk produced by the cow is thus available for sale. Traditionally, cows were expected to lactate for a period of approximately 305 days (see Chapter 6), by which time milk yield would be quite low. They need to be 'dried off' to allow a period of about 60 days (the 'dry period') for regeneration of the udder tissue in preparation for the next lactation. This gives an optimal interval between calvings of one year, and in most intensive systems the practice has been to start re-mating cows between 45 and 60 days postpartum to ensure pregnancy by 80 days after calving, since gestation length is approximately 280–285 days (see Chapter 5). Modern, high genetic dairy cows, especially Holsteins, are capable of producing more milk for longer periods and there are arguments for allowing them longer calving intervals to maximize their potential. Options for calving patterns and intervals are discussed below.

Beef production

Under this system, rather than being separated from the dam shortly after birth, the calf is reared on the cow for the first six months or more of life. This type of production is very widely practised on the American continent, utilizing its extensive ranges. The cow types used were usually based on traditional British beef breeds such as Hereford and Aberdeen Angus, but in recent years European beef breeds (e.g. Belgian Blue, Limousin, Charolais and Simmental) have become more popular. Because of the unpopularity of Holstein calves for beef production, new specialist beef breeds are being developed. For example, the Leachmann Stabilizer is a composite breed made up of four beef breeds (Red Angus, Simmental, Gelbveigh and Hereford). It is naturally polled and is claimed to be hardy and to have easy calving, good calf viability and survival rates, and a very quiet temperament. The resulting females from this dam line programme may be top-crossed with a pure beef bull such as Charolais or Limousin, to give the slaughter generation.

In the single suckler system, the calf remains with its dam and is allowed to suckle ad libitum. In the double and multiple suckler systems, one or more extra calves may be fostered on to the cow. Herds are normally managed with a seasonal calving policy. After weaning, the calves may be further reared on a variety of systems varying from extensive grass/range production to intensive feedlot systems.

Calving patterns and intervals

Before domestication, cows were probably seasonal breeders. Their calving patterns were determined by the availability of the forage on which they relied. In most situations, the breeding season was initiated in the summer, so that calves would be born the following spring, when there was expected to be plenty of fresh pasture and browse available to the cow for milk production to sustain the newborn calf. In non-intensive livestock systems (in the semi-arid tropics, for example) this situation still prevails.

In intensive systems on many beef farms and certain dairy farms, a seasonal calving pattern is adopted as a matter of choice. There are three main possibilities:

- *Spring calving.* This system mimics the natural situation by planning for calving when there is plenty of good quality fodder available relatively cheaply to provide milk for suckling beef calves, or for sale from the dairy herd. Modern, Holstein type, dairy cows may only be able to obtain about half of their milk production needs from grass, and feed management can be difficult. Also, milk prices tend to be lower at this time of year and the system is only viable in areas where there is a long grazing season.
- *Autumn calving.* Cows in early lactation are fed on more expensive conserved forages, with a tendency to greater reliance on concentrate supplementation. If the forage is of known quality this can aid feed management. Rationing can be more precisely controlled and, in the UK at least, cows calving in the autumn produce most of their milk when it is at maximum price. It is advantageous to manage dry cows outside on pasture and, if they are autumn calving, they can then be brought in for optimal management during early and mid lactation.
- *Summer calving.* This system is more difficult to manage, not least because late summer forage tends to be of relatively low and very variable quality. Milk prices tend to be higher in the late summer because of generally low production levels and some farmers choose the system to take advantage of this.

Some cattle farmers, especially in the intensive dairy sector, practise block calving, aiming to calve all their cows within a short period, often as little as two months. One advantage is that tasks such as oestrus detection and insemination and, subsequently, calving and calf care can be concentrated into restricted periods of the year, freeing staff for other tasks, such as silage making and harvesting, at the appropriate time.

As the name suggests, year-round calving herds produce calves throughout the year with, normally, a fairly even spread. This avoids periods of excessive workload and helps to provide regular cash flow. It is relatively easy to manage, accommodating cows with a variety of calving intervals, but, by the same token, reproductive management can become sloppy because cows failing to meet reproductive targets cause fewer problems to the system.

Herd managers may practise variations on, or combinations of, these systems. The herd may, for example, be divided into spring calving and autumn calving sections, whilst on some farms, calving is concentrated into two, or even three, blocks.

As has been said, an annual calving interval has traditionally been a common aim for both beef and dairy producers. It is unrealistic to aim for much shorter intervals, whilst longer intervals were often uneconomic, as cows with extended intervals tend to spend a higher proportion of their existence dry, or producing relatively little milk and fewer calves per year. Some high genetic merit, high yielding cows need more time to conceive, and can be economic at longer intervals, as discussed below.

In some extensive systems in unfavourable climates, where resources are very limited, cows may fail to become pregnant during the breeding season and then lose another year before being capable of conceiving, so that two-year calving intervals are not uncommon, especially in the semi-arid tropics. Some experts maintain that this is a reasonable aim, given the severe environmental and nutritional stresses imposed on the cows. However, lactations tend to be very short, and cows in this situation spend an excessive proportion of their lives non-productively.

High genetic merit Holsteins, for example, producing 8000 litres or more of milk in each lactation, also tend to have more persistent lactations, with flatter lactation curves. It is not unusual for them still to be producing 30–40 litres of milk per day at 305 days. Furthermore, in such cows, conception before 80 days rather than later tends to result in a more severe and lasting depression of yield in mid lactation. Longer calving intervals are easier to achieve in high yielding cows and calf prices are much reduced at the present time, in the UK especially, so there is less economic pressure to produce them as frequently as possible. It has been shown (Wassell *et al.*, 1998) that extending calving intervals by up to three months has no significantly deleterious effect on profitability. There is considerable disagreement on the subject, but the above argument, plus evidence of problems associated with early postpartum insemination of high yielding cows (see Chapter 12), lead us to suggest that intervals of more than 365 days should be accepted, or even actively planned, for them when circumstances permit. Obviously, longer intervals would be impractical in tight seasonal or block calving situations, but if there is more than one calving block, high yielders could be allowed to 'slip back' into later blocks in successive years if they have long calving intervals.

The importance of good reproductive efficiency

Reproduction is a vital factor in determining the efficiency of animal production. At best, a cow is only likely to produce a single calf per year. Therefore bovine reproduction is less efficient than in the other farm species, e.g., pigs and sheep. This also means that the rate of genetic progress is likely to be relatively slow.

In the dairy herd, the goal of ever-increasing milk yields is often pursued to the exclusion of other factors. However, a cow will only begin to lactate effectively after calving and milk yield will eventually cease unless she calves again. Rearing and maintenance costs are high in intensive systems, so that any delay beyond two years to first calving, and any increase in calving interval beyond the optimum, is likely to cause a significant reduction in income. Calves are important both as heifer replacements and for the production of beef. The reproductive process is thus of vital importance.

It has been estimated that sub-fertility results in a financial loss to UK dairy farms alone of up to £500 million per annum. This loss occurs as a result of lost production and higher veterinary, replacement, semen and embryo costs (Lamming *et al.*, 1998). Indeed, the fertility situation is worsening as is discussed below.

Reproductive performance is also closely related to profitability in the beef herd, the most profitable herds having the highest calving rates. The calf is the major product of the herd and so maximum reproductive efficiency is paramount in determining profitability. The calving interval is again a useful measure of fertility, but in suckler herds, for example, calving is usually seasonal, i.e., spring or autumn. In such herds there is an important relationship between the length of the calving season and profitability.

According to a recent Meat and Livestock Commission analysis, the best recorded herds in the UK achieved 75% of cows holding to first service. This means 98% of the cows will calve in 9 weeks and, at weaning, when the oldest calves are 210 days old the entire crop will average 205 days of age. In contrast, the worst herds had a 40% first service pregnancy rate resulting in a 24-week period for 98% of calvings and an equivalent average calf age at weaning of 182 days. At a growth rate of 1 kg/day and a sale price of £1/kg this is a difference of £23/head – or around £18.5 million given the current fertility performance of the UK's 1.4 million suckler cows. On top of this are the extra costs of managing a wider range of calf ages.

A compact calving season is essential for the precise management and feeding of beef cows for a number of reasons:

- More cows calve early in the period; therefore the age and weight of calves are higher at sale. Furthermore, the cows will potentially have a longer interval before they are re-mated and their chances of conception are likely to be greater.
- Calf disease and mortality are likely to be reduced if there is only small variation in calf ages.
- Cows are all at a similar stage in the production cycle, so that they can be regarded as a single unit rather than as individuals and feed can be rationed more precisely.

The calving season is almost directly dependent on the conception rate to service and the length of the breeding (service) period. Obviously the higher the conception rate, the shorter is the service period required to ensure pregnancy of all or the majority of the cows.

The measurement of reproductive efficiency

Reproductive efficiency can be described as a measure of the ability of a cow to become pregnant and produce viable offspring. Infertility or sub-fertility are varying degrees of aberration from typical levels of reproductive performance.

Fertility is usually assessed at the economic level by the calving interval, i.e., the period of time between successive calvings. Historically, British farmers, in common with many others, would aim for the 'ideal' 365-day average interval for their herds. However, a number of cows that have uneconomically short intervals and others with long intervals could contribute to this average, leading to an over optimistic appraisal. Also, as we have seen, it could be desirable to have a longer interval in some cows. The calving interval also fails to take account of those cows that are culled because they have not conceived, or of those cows that have not been served because they have not been detected in oestrus.

From a biological point of view the calving rate is perhaps the most appropriate measure of fertility. This is defined as the number of calves born per 100 services. This also has its drawbacks because it also fails to take account of cows served too long after calving, or never served at all, because of a failure to detect oestrus.

Esslemont (1992) proposed the use of a 'fertility factor', which is the product of the oestrus detection rate and the pregnancy rate (at 45 days post-service). In practice, the oestrus detection rate can be estimated from the submission rate – the percentage of cows inseminated within 23 days of the day they were due for service. The pregnancy rate (the percentage of inseminations that result in a positive pregnancy diagnosis) is then calculated and multiplied by the submission rate to obtain a figure for reproductive efficiency, or the 'fertility factor'. Submission rate should be at least 80% and pregnancy rates should be 70%, giving a figure of 56%. Farmers should be aiming for at least 50%, which contrasts alarmingly with the actual average UK fertility factor of about 20 (48% of 42%; Esslemont & Kossaibati, 2002), having dropped from the figure of 25 calculated by Esslemont (1992).

Esslemont (1992) has also defined a herd fertility economic index (Fertex) score as the cost per cow of extra culling above 22% (£590 per 1%), extended calving intervals over 360 days (£3 per day) and each extra service over two services per conception (£18 per insemination). Esslemont & Peeler (1993) obtained a score of 62 (i.e., a loss of £62 per cow) using the Dairy Information System (DAISY), University of Reading, to interpret actual fertility data from 91 UK dairy herds. In 2003, the figure was £183 (Esslemont, 2003).

Components of the calving interval

The calving interval can be divided into two components:

(1) *The calving to conception interval.* This is the time from parturition until the establishment of the next pregnancy. It is this interval that is the main determinant of the calving interval, and is thus the parameter that is usually manipulated in order to try to achieve the target calving interval.

(2) *The gestation period.* This is normally between 280 and 285 days in the cow, the variation being mainly due to genetic influences of both the dam and the sire. It can be shortened to only a limited degree by the artificial induction of parturition (see Chapter 6).

Factors affecting the calving to conception interval

In order to achieve a 365-day calving interval the calving to conception interval should not be more than 80–85 days. For the purpose of recording reproductive performance on the farm the calving to conception interval is often subdivided into two components: the calving to first service interval and the first service to conception interval.

The calving to first service interval depends on (1) the re-establishment of ovarian cycles after calving, (2) the occurrence and detection of oestrus and (3) the herdsperson's planned start of services date, if this is later than (1) and (2).

The first service to conception interval is dependent on (1) the ability to conceive and maintain pregnancy after a given service and (2) the continuation of ovarian cycles and the correct detection of oestrus in those cows that do not conceive to initial services. The interrelationships of the above parameters with blood or milk concentrations of the ovarian hormone progesterone are illustrated in Fig. 1.1.

All of these parameters, except for the planned start of service date, depend on a combination of genotypic and environmental factors affecting the cows. The ability to conceive also depends on the fertility of the semen used at a particular insemination and the effectiveness of the insemination procedure.

Esslemont & Ellis (1974) showed that the calving to first service interval and the first service to conception interval are dependent on both the oestrus detection rate and the average conception rate in the herd. Examples of the relationships between components of the calving to conception interval are given in Table 1.3 for oestrus detection rates of 50% and 80% and illustrate the way in which such information can be used to analyse the causes of poor reproductive performance in herds so that appropriate corrective measures can be applied. For example, if a herd's calving to first service interval is 65 days, the average conception rate is 60% and if the calving to conception interval is 93 days, this indicates that the oestrus detection rate is only 50%. Therefore, more attention to the detection of oestrus (see Chapter 8) so that 80% of oestrous periods are detected would reduce the average calving to conception interval to around 82 days, close to that required for a 365-day calving interval.

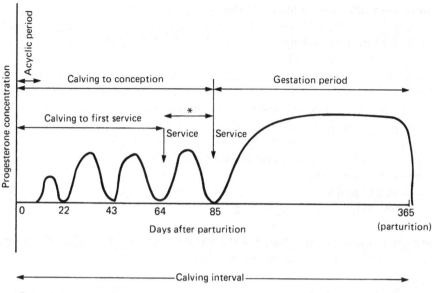

Fig. 1.1 Relationship of progesterone concentrations to the calving interval and its components.

Table 1.3 The effect of mean interval to first service, conception rate and oestrus detection rate on mean calving to conception intervals. (From Esslemont & Ellis, 1974.)

Mean interval from calving to first service (days)	Calving to conception interval									
	At 80% oestrus detection rate					At 50% oestrus detection rate				
	Average conception rate (%)					Average conception rate (%)				
	40	45	50	55	60	40	45	50	55	60
50	87	80	76	71	67	110	98	92	84	78
55	92	85	81	76	72	115	103	97	89	83
60	97	90	86	81	77	120	108	102	94	88
65	102	95	91	86	82	125	113	107	99	93
70	107	100	96	91	87	130	118	112	104	98
75	112	105	101	96	92	135	123	117	109	103
80	117	110	106	101	97	140	128	122	114	108
85	122	115	111	106	102	145	133	127	119	113
90	127	120	116	111	107	150	138	132	124	118
95	132	125	121	116	112	155	143	137	129	123

In practice it can be extremely difficult to determine the causes of extended calving intervals. If, for example, the calving to first service interval is extended because oestrus was not detected, this could be due to either:

• a failure of the cow to exhibit oestrus or
• a failure of the stockperson to detect oestrus.

Failure to exhibit oestrus might be due to:

- a lack of ovarian activity
- abnormal ovarian activity or
- a 'silent ovulation', i.e., ovulation unaccompanied by oestrous behaviour.

Also, if a cow is observed in oestrus more than one cycle length (21 days) after service, this could be due to:

- an intervening oestrous period having been missed
- abnormal cycle length
- loss of a conceptus
- oestrus occurring during pregnancy.

Similarly, if a cow is inseminated at the wrong time (i.e., not within about one day of ovulation), this could be due to either:

- stockperson error or
- the cow showing oestrous symptoms at the wrong time. She may or may not be suffering from an ovarian abnormality which would interfere with normal fertility.

Thus the clinician is often faced with a difficult task in trying to unravel the causes of poor reproductive performance.

Reproductive expectancy

Even under ideal conditions, with 100% 'normal' cows and 100% efficiency of oestrus detection, calving rates will fail to reach 100%. At best, only 60–70% of inseminations in cows result in a calf being born, with a large majority of the failures occurring before the second trimester of pregnancy. This is due in part to conception failure and in part to embryonic or fetal death (see Chapter 12), both of which occur in most species. Under experimental conditions, fertilization rates in cows, as assessed by examination of ova and embryos after slaughter or surgery, have been estimated to be in excess of 90%, although the figure may well be lower under normal farm conditions. Nevertheless, a high proportion of reproductive failure apparently results from embryonic or fetal death. It was suggested by Bishop (1964) that the majority of embryonic/fetal mortality occurs because of genetic abnormalities in the embryos, as a result of which they are eliminated at 'a low biological cost'. This suggests that such losses are inevitable even in normal fertile cows and that attempts to prevent them would be ineffective and even undesirable. However, this hypothesis has never been conclusively demonstrated.

Table 1.4 Reproductive expectation for 100 cows each with a 60% probability of calving to each service.

Order no. of insemination	No. of inseminations	No. of calves born	No. of returns to service
1	100	60	40
2	40	24	16
3	16	9.6	6.4
4	6.4	3.8	2.6
5	2.6	1.6	1.0
Total	165	99	—

Table 1.5 Theoretical calving interval for cows with a 60% probability of calving to each service. (From David *et al.*, 1971.)

	Days
Mean gestation period	280
Mean interval from calving to first service[a]	70
Mean interval required for re-insemination ($0.65^b \times 21^c$)	14
Mean theoretical calving interval	365

[a] Assuming the recommendation of serving at the first oestrus after calving is followed.
[b] The average number of extra inseminations required per calf born at 60% calving rate.
[c] The length of one oestrus cycle. This is likely to be an optimistic figure, even assuming all returns are detected as soon as they occur, since more than 10% of cows are likely to suffer from early fetal loss more than 21 days after service (see Ball, 1997).

Table 1.4 shows the expected reproductive performance of a herd of 100 cows that has a 60% calving rate. This means that 60% of all first services, 60% of all second services, and so on, will result in full-term pregnancies. The result is that, simply by chance, 6.4% of the cows will need four or more services to achieve successful pregnancy, even though there is no detectable abnormality. This means that, on average, 1.65 inseminations are required per calf born. Even at 70% calving rate, 2.7% of cows will need four or more services. This figure has been used as the basis of the theoretical calculation of calving interval shown in Table 1.5. This shows that even in the absence of specific fertility problems it is difficult to achieve the 'ideal' 365-day calving interval.

All this does not mean of course that calving rates will never achieve 100%. Clearly there must be a specific cause(s) for almost 50% of services to fail. The cause is likely to be multifactorial, involving an interaction between genetics and environment/management. This is currently a hotly debated issue in relation to declining dairy cow fertility.

To summarize, in this introductory chapter we have attempted to explain the importance of reproductive efficiency in relation to cattle production systems and to highlight the following points:

- Reproductive performance is crucial in determining the efficiency of a breeding cattle enterprise, but is generally well below the level considered optimal and practically feasible.
- Recording of fertility is complex, but various parameters can be used to quantify reproductive performance.
- In the present state of knowledge 100% reproductive efficiency cannot be achieved and appears to be declining in some sectors.

Future chapters will expand the various concepts introduced in this one, with the aim of providing a comprehensive account of the physiological and management factors that combine to determine reproductive efficiency in a breeding herd.

References

Ball, P.J.H. (1997) *Animal Breeding Abstracts*, **65**, 167–175 (Review).

Bishop, M.W.H. (1964) *Journal of Reproduction and Fertility*, **7**, 383.

David, J.S.E., Bishop, M.W.H. & Cembrowicz, H.J. (1971) *Veterinary Record*, **89**, 181.

Esslemont, R.J. (1992) *Veterinary Record*, **131**, 209.

Esslemont, R.J. (2003) *Proceedings of BCVA and Dutch Cattle Veterinary Association Joint Conference on Fertility*, Amsterdam, October.

Esslemont, R.J. & Ellis, P.R. (1974) *Veterinary Record*, 5 Oct, 319.

Esslemont, R.J. & Kossaibati, M.A. (2002) *Daisy Report No. 5*.

Esslemont, R.J. & Peeler, P.R. (1993) *British Veterinary Journal*, **149**, 537–547.

Lamming, G.E., Darwash, A.O., Wathes, D.C. & Ball, P.J.H. (1998) *Journal of the Royal Agricultural Society of England*, **159**, 82–93.

National Dairy Council (2002) *Dairy Facts and Figures*.

Wassell, T.R., Stott, A.W. & Wassell, B.R. (1998) *Proceedings of the 49th Annual Meeting of the European Association of Animal Production*, Warsaw.

Chapter 2
Anatomy

The male reproductive tract consists of testes, penis and accessory organs and is designed to produce the male gametes (spermatozoa) and introduce them into the female reproductive tract. The latter includes (1) the ovaries, which produce the female gametes (oocytes), (2) the oviducts, which provide a site for the union of the male and female gametes at fertilization, and (3) the uterus, where the resulting conceptus develops.

The male and female genitalia are both derived from identical tissue in the early embryo. The ovaries and testes arise from a common origin in the region of the developing kidney. They begin to become recognizable at about 7–8 weeks of gestation. Both structures change their position during fetal life, the testes migrating further than the ovaries. Both ovaries and testes are normally in the adult position at the time of birth.

The tubular genitalia are formed from two sets of longitudinal ducts, which develop simultaneously in the embryo. In the male, the Wolffian ducts eventually differentiate into the efferent ducts, epididymes and vasa deferentia, while in the female the Müllerian ducts develop into the oviducts, uterus, cervix and anterior vagina.

The genitalia in the male and in the female are ultimately under the endocrine control of the same structures, i.e., the hypothalamus and the pituitary gland.

Organs controlling male and female genitalia

The hypothalamus

The hypothalamus lies at the base of the brainstem just posterior to the point at which the optic nerves enter, forming the optic chiasma (Fig. 2.1). Histologically it consists of several discrete masses of nerve cell bodies or nuclei of which the paraventricular nucleus, supraoptic nucleus and the median eminence are the most distinct (Fig. 2.2). The hypothalamus is involved in the control of physiological processes as diverse as temperature regulation, appetite and reactions such as fear and rage, in addition to the control of the function of the pituitary gland.

The activity of the hypothalamus is controlled by numerous neural connections from higher brain centres. Those higher brain centres involved in the control of reproduction assume varying importance in different species but in general include the olfactory bulbs responsible for the sense of smell, the

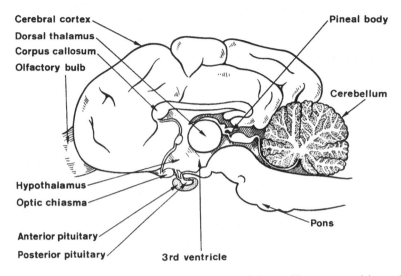

Fig. 2.1 Diagrammatic midline section of the brain to illustrate position of the hypothalamus and pituitary gland.

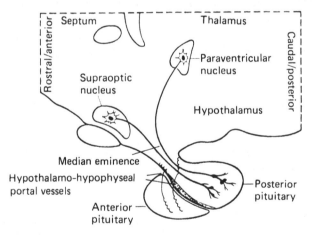

Fig. 2.2 The hypothalamus and pituitary gland, illustrating the vascular connection between the hypothalamus and anterior pituitary and neural connection between the hypothalamus and posterior pituitary.

cerebral cortex which processes visual and auditory stimuli and the pineal body which is thought to mediate effects of other environmental stimuli such as photoperiod (Fig. 2.1).

The hypothalamic releasing factor gonadotrophin releasing hormone (GnRH) [alternatively called luteinizing hormone releasing hormone (LHRH)] is a polypeptide consisting of ten amino acid residues (see Fig. 2.3).

Pyroglutamate–histidine–tryptophan–serine–tyrosine–glycine–leucine–arginine–proline–glycine

Fig. 2.3 Molecular structure of gonadotrophin releasing hormone (GnRH). (From Matsuo *et al.*, 1971a.)

Injection of cattle with GnRH causes a dose-dependent release of both luteinizing hormone (LH) and follicle stimulating hormone (FSH). It is currently accepted that the single decapeptide GnRH is responsible for both LH and FSH secretion, although the responsiveness of each type of gonadotrophin cell in the anterior pituitary gland is able to vary differentially with the stage of the oestrous cycle. The pattern of GnRH secretion during the oestrous cycle has not been characterized in cows due to difficulties in its measurement in peripheral blood. However, a clear relationship between GnRH release and LH release has been established in other species and is no doubt similar in cattle.

The hypothalamus also secretes thyrotrophin releasing hormone (TRH), a tripeptide which stimulates the release of thyroid stimulating hormone (TSH) and prolactin from the anterior pituitary, and prolactin inhibiting factor (PIF).

The pituitary gland

The pituitary gland or hypophysis lies at the base of the forebrain below the hypothalamus and consists of anterior and posterior parts (Figs 2.1 and 2.2). The anterior pituitary gland or adenohypophysis consists of true glandular tissue and, although attached to the brainstem, is derived embryologically from an evagination in the roof of the oral cavity known as Rathke's pouch. The posterior pituitary gland or neurohypophysis is composed of specialized neural or neurosecretory tissue and is derived embryologically from the developing brainstem.

The anterior pituitary gland

The anterior pituitary gland secretes several hormones, all large molecular weight proteins that control various functions in the body. These include:

- Follicle stimulating hormone (FSH): a glycoprotein with a molecular weight of approximately 25000. It consists of two protein fractions, the α-subunit and the β-subunit. This hormone may be regarded as the initiator of ovarian activity since it directly promotes growth of ovarian follicles.
- Luteinizing hormone (LH): a glycoprotein with a molecular weight of approximately 40000. It also consists of an α-subunit and the β-subunit, the former being identical to that of FSH. The function of LH appears to be primarily to stimulate the maturation and ovulation of the antral follicle and secondly to stimulate the formation and maintenance of the corpus luteum.

- Prolactin: a protein hormone of molecular weight approximately 23 000. It is gonadotrophic in some species, but does not appear to have this role in the cow.
- Growth hormone (GH).
- Thyroid stimulating hormone (TSH).
- Adrenocorticotrophic hormone (ACTH).

The anterior pituitary gland synthesizes and secretes hormones in response to 'releasing hormones', which are secreted by the hypothalamus. These reach the cells of the anterior pituitary via the hypothalamo-hypophyseal portal blood vessels which originate mainly in the area of the median eminence (Fig. 2.2), thus stimulating the release of anterior pituitary hormones.

The posterior pituitary gland

The posterior pituitary gland secretes two peptide hormones, oxytocin and vasopressin. These hormones are synthesized in the paraventricular and supraoptic nuclei of the hypothalamus and droplets pass down the axons of specialized secretory neurones into the posterior pituitary gland (Fig. 2.2) from where they are secreted into the systemic circulation.

The male reproductive tract

The male reproductive tract consists of primary, secondary and accessory sex organs. The primary male sex organs are the testes, which are located in the scrotum suspended externally in the inguinal region. The secondary sex organs consist of the duct tissues, which transport sperm from the testes to the exterior and include the efferent ducts within the testes, epididymes, vasa deferentia, the penis and the urethra. The accessory organs consist of the prostate gland, the seminal vesicles and the bulbo-urethral (Cowper's) glands. The anatomical relationship of these organs is shown in Fig. 2.4.

The testes

Production of spermatozoa requires temperatures below that of the body and a system has evolved such that the testes are maintained in the scrotum outside the body wall. The scrotum is lined internally by muscle, the dartos tunic, which can contract to pull the scrotum closer to the body wall in cold weather and vice versa in a warm environment. Testicular size in the adult bull is variable but averages 10–12 cm in length and 6–8 cm in diameter. The testes stand upright in the scrotum with the epididymis lying closely apposed to the posterior surface (Fig. 2.4).

Each testis is suspended by a spermatic cord, which contains the blood supply (internal spermatic artery) and venous drainage (spermatic vein) in the

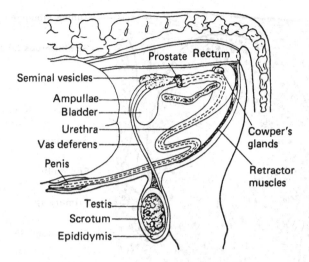

Fig. 2.4 The reproductive tract of the bull (lateral view).

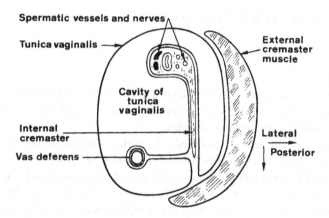

Fig. 2.5 Transverse section of the spermatic cord of the bull. (From Sisson & Grossman, 1967.)

anterior portion and the vas deferens in the posterior portion (Fig. 2.5). The venous drainage forms the pampiniform plexus in the base of the cord, a complex network of veins around the spermatic artery, which serves to cool the arterial blood before it reaches the testicular tissue. The base of the testis is anchored in the scrotum by the scrotal ligament. Each testis is surrounded by the tunica vaginalis, which is a continuation of the peritoneum (the membrane lining the abdominal cavity) and consists of two layers of fibrous membrane. The outer layer lines the internal surface of the scrotum whilst the inner layer covers the spermatic cord, testis and epididymis. The external cremaster muscle, by which the testes can be raised towards the body wall, lies on the

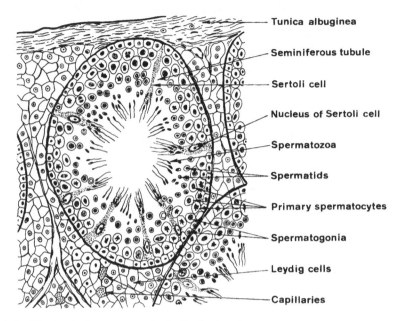

Tunica albuginea

Seminiferous tubule

Sertoli cell

Nucleus of Sertoli cell

Spermatozoa

Spermatids

Primary spermatocytes

Spermatogonia

Leydig cells

Capillaries

Fig. 2.6 Histological structure of a testicular lobule.

lateral-posterior side of the spermatic cord (Fig. 2.5). The spermatic cord enters the abdominal cavity through the inguinal canal, a ring formed between the bony pelvis and the abdominal muscles.

The interior of the testis is divided into compartments or lobules by tough fibrous membranes or septa. Each lobule consists of up to four seminiferous tubules embedded in stromal tissue consisting of blood vessels, nerves and the so-called Leydig cells (Fig. 2.6). Each tubule is highly convoluted and is 30–70 cm long and 0.2 mm in diameter. The tubule is lined by the seminiferous cells which are of two types: the spermatogenic cells or spermatogonia, which give rise to spermatozoa; and the Sertoli cells which supply nutrients to the spermatogonia.

Expression of genes on the Y chromosome of the male fetus programmes the undifferentiated gonad to form a testicle rather than an ovary. Testicular function is initiated quite early in fetal life and is responsible for the development of the male reproductive tract and suppression of development of the female tract. Development of the male tract is initiated and maintained by testosterone secretion from the Leydig cells, beginning as early as day 42 of gestation. Castration of a bovine male fetus before day 40 of pregnancy would result in the birth of a phenotypic female. Development of the female tract is suppressed by a hormonal factor secreted by the Sertoli cells (Josso *et al.*, 1979). Final testicular development and descent into the scrotum occurs long before birth in cattle, sheep and pigs.

The functions of the testes are twofold: (1) the secretion of testosterone and other steroid hormones by the Leydig cells, and (2) production of spermatozoa (spermatogenesis). Spermatogenesis, the production of spermatozoa, is described in Chapter 3.

Secondary male sex organs

The lumina of the testicular tubules communicate with the epididymis via the efferent ducts. The passage of spermatozoa through the epididymis involves their maturation, which includes completion of differentiation and acquisition of their own mobility. The vas deferens which carries spermatozoa from the epididymis to the urethra passes up through the spermatic cord to join the urethra near the neck of the urinary bladder (Fig. 2.4). The urethra arises at the neck of the bladder and extends to the outside through the penis. It is the common route of exit for both urine and semen.

The penis consists of three parts, the root, the body and the glans penis, the latter being the free end. The root and posterior part of the body are attached to the bony pelvis by a system of ligaments and muscles (Fig. 2.7). The penis is cylindrical and composed mainly of erectile tissue, a network of channels which become engorged with blood during arousal. This causes the penis to enlarge and to be extruded. Just behind the scrotum, the penis forms an S-shaped curve, the sigmoid flexure, which is straightened during erection. The glans penis forms the anterior 8 cm or so of the penis and normally lies within the sheath

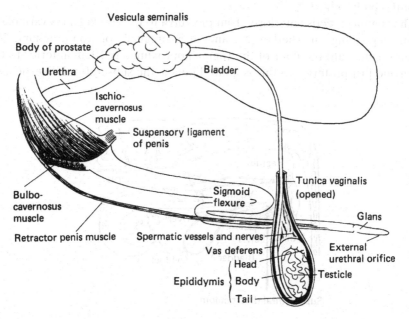

Fig. 2.7   The reproductive system of the bull, illustrating muscle attachments of the penis. (Redrawn from Sisson & Grossman, 1967.)

or prepuce. During erection the penis may be extruded up to 55 cm from the prepuce.

Accessory male sex organs (Fig. 2.4)

The prostate gland is small and lies above the neck of the bladder close to the origin of the urethra. The paired seminal vesicles are lobulated, 10–12 cm in length, approximately 5 cm in width and lie on either side of the neck of the bladder close to the prostate. The bulbo-urethral glands measure approximately 2.5 × 1 cm and lie on either side of the urethra, approximately 10 cm behind the prostate. These accessory male glands secrete specific components of seminal plasma (Chapter 3).

The female reproductive tract

The female genitalia lie in the pelvic cavity and consist of the vulva, vagina, cervix, uterus, fallopian tubes, ovaries and supporting structures (see Fig. 2.8).

The vulva and vagina

The vulva, or lips, form the exterior opening of the reproductive tract and allow for the entry of the bull's penis (or the AI gun) at service and for the expulsion of the calf at birth. In the cow, the vulva also forms the exit point of urine from the body (Fig. 2.9).

The vagina extends anteriorly from the vulva to the cervix and is variable in length depending on whether the animal is pregnant or non-pregnant. The urethra opens into the floor of the vagina approximately 10 cm anterior to the vulva and just posterior to this is a blind pouch, the sub-urethral diverticulum

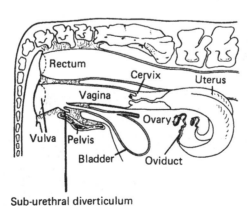

Fig. 2.8   The reproductive tract of the cow (lateral view), showing its position inside the pelvic and abdominal cavities.

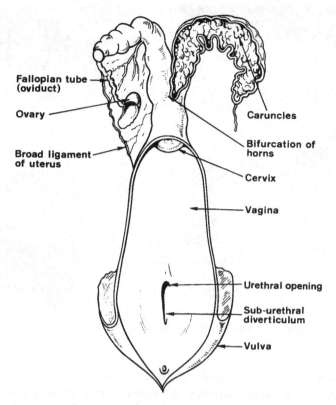

Fallopian tube (oviduct)

Ovary

Broad ligament of uterus

Caruncles

Bifurcation of horns

Cervix

Vagina

Urethral opening

Sub-urethral diverticulum

Vulva

Fig. 2.9 Dorsal view of the reproductive tract of the cow. The vagina and right horn of the uterus have been opened.

(Figs 2.8 and 2.9). The vaginal wall is tough and elastic and the lining or epithelium changes with the stage of the oestrous cycle. The cells near to the cervix produce mucus and are particularly active around the time of oestrus.

The cervix

Commonly known as the neck of the womb, the cervix forms a barrier between the vagina and uterus. It varies in length from 2–3 cm in the heifer to approximately 10 cm in the mature cow and has a very thick fibrous wall. The lumen or cervical canal is convoluted and normally tightly closed except at parturition, although it also dilates slightly at oestrus. A plug of thick brownish mucus is usually present in the canal during the luteal phase of the cycle and during pregnancy.

The uterus

The uterus is a hollow muscular organ consisting of a short body and two relatively long cornua or horns. Thus when straightened the tract is Y-shaped,

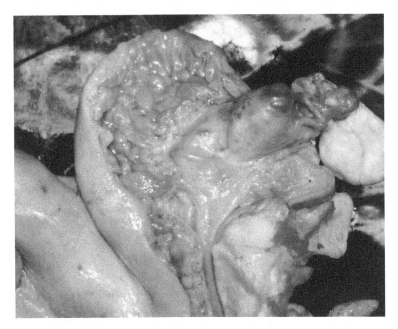

Fig. 2.10   Uterine horn of a heifer opened to show the caruncles.

although in life the uterine horns curve downwards and laterally (Figs 2.8 and 2.9). The size of the uterus depends on factors such as age and parity, but the uterine body is approximately 5 cm in length and the horns are 20–40 cm in length and 1.5–4 cm in external diameter in the non-pregnant cow, tapering at the ovarian extremity. Of course, during pregnancy the uterus increases in size and this is discussed in detail in Chapter 5. The uterus is suspended in the pelvic cavity by the broad uterine ligaments on either side. These ligaments also carry the blood and nerve supply to the tract. Blood is supplied to the tract by the utero-ovarian and uterine arteries of which the middle uterine artery is the largest.

The uterine wall varies from 3–10 mm in thickness and consists of three layers: the inner lining or endometrium; a muscular layer, the myometrium; and the outer 'serosa' layer. The endometrium or mucosa consists mainly of glandular epithelium and has approximately 120 specialized raised areas known as 'caruncles' (Figs 2.9 and 2.10). These are characteristic of the uterus of ruminants and are the points of attachment of the placenta during pregnancy (see Chapter 5).

The fallopian tubes

The fallopian tubes or oviducts serve to transport ova or unfertilized eggs from the ovary to the uterus and pursue a convoluted course through a section of the broad ligament, the mesosalpinx. Each oviduct is 20–30 cm long and

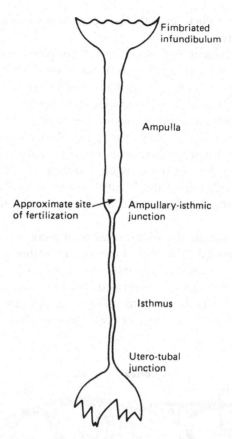

Fig. 2.11 Schematic diagram of a fallopian tube or oviduct. (From Hunter, 1980.)

approximately 2–3 mm in diameter and can be considered as consisting of three segments (Fig. 2.11).

The narrow isthmus extends from the tip of the uterine horn for about half the length of the oviduct; the ampulla is a slightly wider section eventually opening into the peritoneal cavity via the funnel-like third portion or infundibulum. This acts literally as a funnel, which serves to capture ova as they are shed from the ovary at ovulation and to facilitate their passage down the oviduct.

The ovaries

The two ovaries lie slightly medially to the tips of the uterine horns to which they are joined directly by parts of the broad ligaments, the ovarian ligament. They are oval in shape and vary in size from about 1.5–5 cm in length and 1–3 cm in diameter, depending on the stage of reproductive cycle. Ovarian structure is not static, and the appearance of the surface of the ovary continually changes in cycles of follicle growth and regression or ovulation and corpus luteum growth and regression.

Oogenesis, the production of ova or eggs, takes place from a group of cells, the oogonia, which develop in cords from the germinal epithelium surrounding the fetal ovary. These cells penetrate the ovarian stroma and gradually differentiate, the larger ones eventually becoming the primary oocytes or egg cells. The neighbouring cells surround the oocyte and provide sustenance, the whole structure being known as a primary ovarian follicle. Each female animal has a full complement of primary follicles containing primary oocytes at birth, but the number is far in excess of those required during life. The primary follicles enter phases of growth during the lifetime of the animal, a process possibly under hormonal control, although the precise nature of the stimulus is not understood.

In the immature female the ovary consists of a cortex containing primary oocytes, each surrounded by a single layer of supporting cells, and a medulla containing connective tissue, nerves and blood vessels (Fig. 2.12).

The growth of follicles is controlled by the neuroendocrine system. During follicular growth, the cells surrounding the primary oocyte increase in number thus increasing the number of layers around the cell. With continued

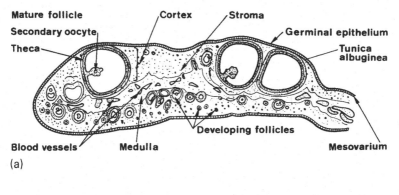

(a)

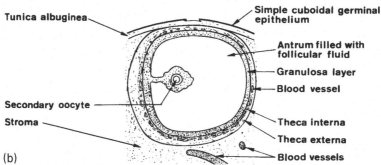

(b)

Fig. 2.12 (a) Longitudinal section of an ovary and (b) section through an ovarian follicle. (From Freeman & Bracegirdle, 1968.)

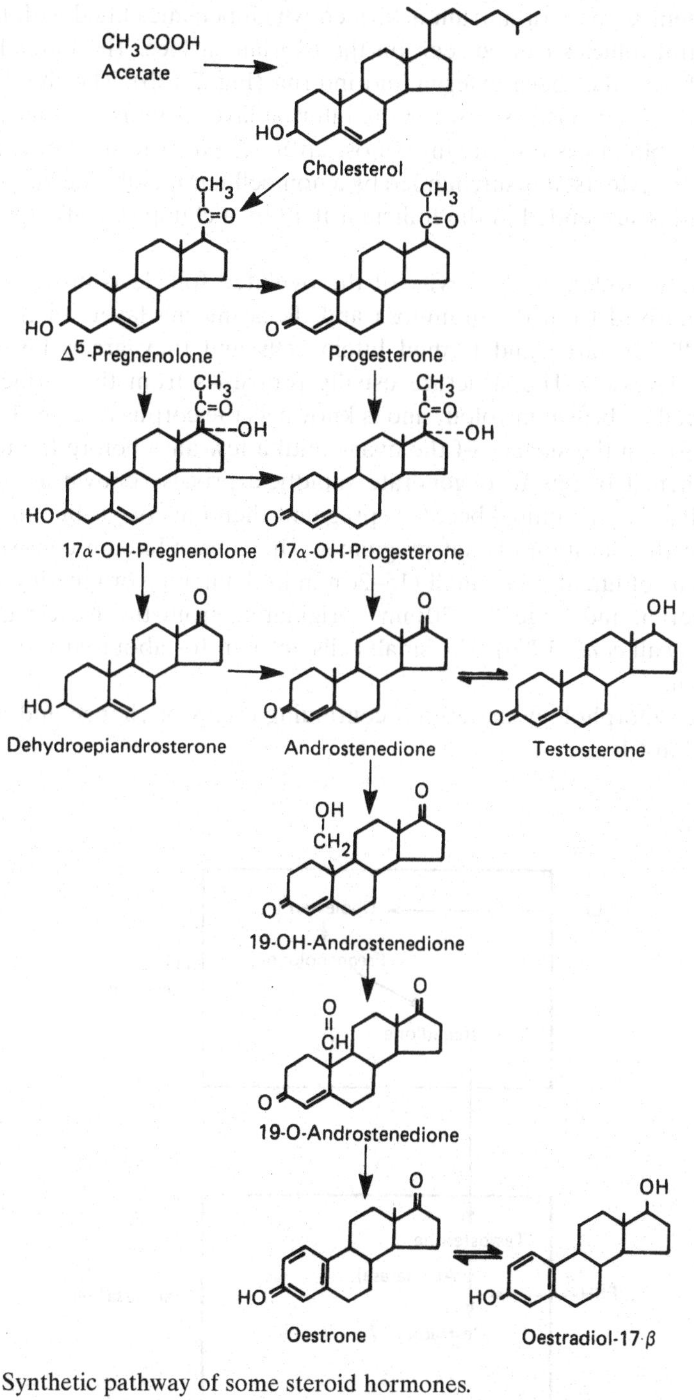

Fig. 2.13   Synthetic pathway of some steroid hormones.

development a cavity or antrum is formed which becomes filled with follicular fluid. Antral follicles can be seen on the ovarian surface. The outer layers of the follicle are the theca externa and interna (Fig. 2.12b). The theca externa contains much fibrous tissue while the internal layer is more cellular and contains many blood vessels. The innermost layer of cells is termed the granulosa layer. The oocyte itself is surrounded by a non-cellular membrane, the zona pellucida, and is suspended in the follicular fluid by a clump of cells, the cumulus oophorus.

Following ovulation, the cavity of the ovulated follicle is invaded by cells that are derived from the granulosa and theca interna layers of the follicle. These cells are large and termed lutein cells and they are richly supplied with blood vessels. The structure usually protrudes from the surface of the ovary, is yellow-brown in colour and is known as the corpus luteum. This structure persists on the surface of the ovary until a few days before the next ovulation, when it begins to degenerate rapidly, a process known as luteolysis. Alternatively if the animal becomes pregnant then the corpus luteum is maintained for the duration of that pregnancy. The corpus luteum consists of two populations of luteal cells: small (15–20 mm in diameter), originating from the theca interna, and large (25–30 mm), originating from the follicle granulosa layer (Schwall *et al.*, 1986). The small cells account for about 90% of the total population.

Ovarian morphology undergoes continuing cycles of change and these are described in Chapter 4.

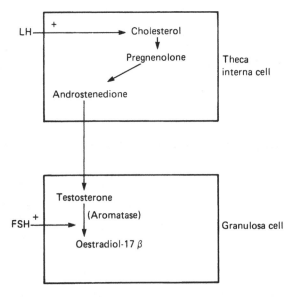

Fig. 2.14 Schematic representation of the synthetic pathway of oestradiol-17β in ovarian follicles. (Adapted from Hansel and Convey, 1983.)

Various steroid hormones are secreted by the bovine ovary, the most important of these being the oestrogens and progesterone. All steroids are synthesized from cholesterol which is in turn produced from acetate inside the cell, or alternatively taken up from the blood. The synthetic pathways for the steroid hormones are shown in Fig. 2.13.

The principal biologically active oestrogen is oestradiol-17β; the others, oestriol and oestrone, may be considered as metabolites of oestradiol. Both the theca interna and granulosa layers of the follicle are involved in oestrogen synthesis. Testosterone is synthesized from cholesterol, the common steroid precursor, in the theca interna under the control of LH and FSH. Testosterone is then converted to oestradiol-17β in the granulosa cells by the action of the enzyme aromatase (Fig. 2.14). Oestradiol is then secreted into the fluid of developing antral follicles and into the ovarian veins.

Both small and large cells in the corpus luteum secrete progesterone. The small cells are very sensitive to LH whilst the large cells are more responsive to prostaglandin E (Hansel *et al.*, 1991). The large cells are also thought to be the source of luteal oxytocin.

References

Freeman, W.H. & Bracegirdle, B. (1968) *An Atlas of Histology.* Heinemann, London.

Hansel, W. & Convey, E.M. (1983) *Journal of Animal Science*, **57** (Suppl. 2), 404.

Hansel, W., Alila, H.W., Dowd, J.P. & Milvae, R.A. (1991) *Journal of Reproduction and Fertility* (Suppl. 43), 77.

Hunter, R.H.F. (1980) *Physiology and Technology of Reproduction in Female Domestic Animals.* Academic Press, London.

Josso, N.J., Picard, Y., Dacheux, J.L. & Courot, M. (1979) *Journal of Reproduction and Fertility*, **57**, 397.

Matsuo, H., Arimura, A., Nair, R.M.G. & Schally, A.V. (1971a) *Biochemical and Biophysical Research Communications*, **45**, 822.

Schwall, R.H., Sawyer, H.R. & Niswender, G.D. (1986) *Journal of Reproduction and Fertility*, **76**, 821.

Sisson, S. & Grossman, J.D. (1967) *The Anatomy of the Domestic Animals*, 4th edn. W.B. Saunders, Philadelphia.

Chapter 3
Bull Fertility

Bulls are used either to serve cows naturally or as donors of semen for use in artificial insemination (AI). In the case of natural service, a single bull may be expected to serve a herd of up to 60 or more cows. On the other hand, the use of a bull for AI may mean that a large number of doses of semen could be prepared from each ejaculate. Therefore the fertility or reproductive capacity of the individual bull is a crucial factor in determining the reproductive performance of cows, i.e., a plentiful supply of normal spermatozoa is essential, as is the sexual desire (libido) which ultimately leads to the ejaculation of the spermatozoa into a real or artificial vagina. Unfortunately the fertility of bulls used for natural service is rarely investigated and this can lead to substantial and expensive delay in the discovery of fertility problems. The present chapter discusses the bull's normal reproductive function and its physiological control.

Puberty

In general, puberty in the bull occurs when the bull calf first produces sufficient sperm to successfully impregnate a female. This has been more pragmatically defined as the time when a bull first produces an ejaculate containing 50 million sperm of which more than 10% are motile (Wolf *et al.*, 1965). The pubertal period is associated with rapid testicular growth, changes in the LH release pattern, an increase in blood plasma testosterone concentrations and the initiation of spermatogenesis.

Stages of testicular development were defined by Fossland & Schultz (1961) for dairy-type bulls, and a summary of their classification is shown below:

Stage 1 Neonatal development and lumenization of tubules and appearance of spermatocytes.
Stage 2 Prepubertal appearance of secondary spermatocytes and spermatids.
Stage 3 Circumpubertal appearance of spermatozoa in the testis and epididymis.
Stage 4 Postpubertal hyperplasia of testicular tissue.

A variety of factors influence the age at which puberty is reached, via effects on the neuroendocrine system. The most important of these are breed, energy intake, liveweight gain and season of birth. Puberty usually occurs in the bull between seven and nine months of age. First sexual interest may coincide with the development of fertilizing capacity or may precede it by a variable period. Although bulls are fertile during the immediate postpubertal period, semen volume, total number of spermatozoa and number of motile spermatozoa all increase over subsequent months as does fertility determined by non-return rate.

Testicular function

The two main functions of the testes (the secretion of testosterone and other steroid hormones by the Leydig cells, and the production of spermatozoa) are controlled mainly by hormones from the anterior pituitary gland. The secretion of testosterone, which is responsible for the bull's libido, is controlled by the action of luteinizing hormone (LH), sometimes known as interstitial cell-stimulating hormone (ICSH) in the male.

The rate of LH secretion increases during the first few weeks after birth, attaining a high level between two and five months of age. Plasma LH concentrations then fall to approximately those of the early postnatal period. The fall in the concentrations appears to coincide with an increase in testosterone secretion, which exerts a 'negative feedback' effect on LH, thereby suppressing its secretion. Both LH and testosterone are secreted as discrete episodes or pulses, the amplitude and frequency of which determine the average plasma concentrations of that hormone (Fig. 3.1).

As testosterone secretion develops, each pulse of LH is followed approximately one hour later by a pulse of testosterone secretion (Schams *et al.*, 1978) and the magnitude of the testosterone response increases with age (Rawlings *et al.*, 1978). This increase in testosterone response is thought to augment the

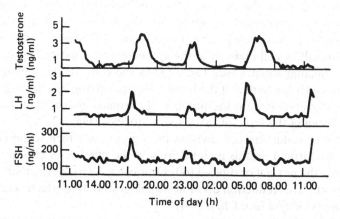

Fig. 3.1 Short-term changes in concentrations of testosterone, LH and FSH in peripheral blood plasma of a bull. (From Schams *et al.*, 1981.)

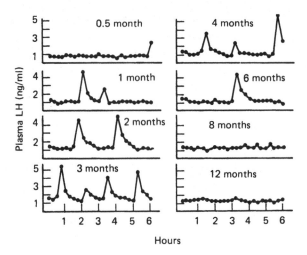

Fig. 3.2 Changes in the pattern of LH secretion in a bull calf from two weeks of age up to 12 months. Note the increase in LH pulse frequency over the first 3–4 months, followed by a decrease in frequency. (From Pelletier *et al.*, 1981.)

negative feedback effect on LH secretion, resulting in the fall in LH secretion observed after five months of age (Pelletier *et al.*, 1981). Changes in LH pulse frequency in prepubertal bulls are illustrated in Fig. 3.2.

Plasma concentrations of FSH appear to change little during the prepubertal period although it does appear to be secreted in pulses synchronous with those of LH (see Fig. 3.1). Once puberty is reached, pulsatile releases of pituitary LH continue to stimulate the Leydig cells to produce testosterone, high levels of which exert a negative feedback effect on the hypothalamus, suppressing GnRH and thus LH production. Testosterone is also involved in sperm (spermatozoon) production through its action on the Sertoli cells (see below).

Spermatogenesis, or the process of sperm (spermatozoon) production, is composed of two processes: spermatocytogenesis and spermiogenesis. Spermatocytogenesis is the development of spermatogenic tissue in the testis, which occurs as a result of cell division of the spermatogonia, located at the periphery of the testicular lobules (see Fig. 2.6). As the cells divide they move progressively towards the lumen of the lobule. The spermatogonia undergo several mitotic cell divisions (where the number of chromosomes remain the same), eventually forming the large primary spermatocytes (Fig. 3.3).

A meiotic or reduction cell division then occurs in which secondary spermatocytes are formed. In this meiotic division the number of chromosomes is reduced from the normal or diploid (60 chromosomes) to the haploid (30 chromosomes) state. This reduction division is analogous to that which occurs in the female primary oocyte (see Chapter 4).

After the meiotic division of the primary spermatocytes, the secondary spermatocytes divide further to form smaller cells, the spermatids (Fig. 3.3). Each

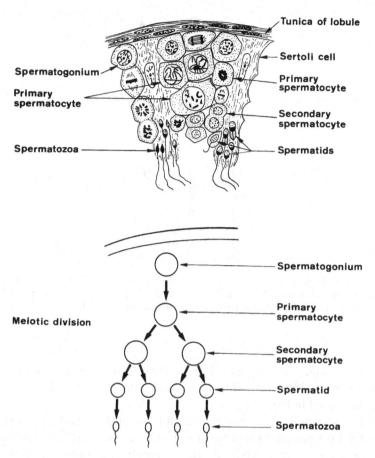

Fig. 3.3 Production of spermatozoa.

secondary spermatocyte produces two spermatids. During the subsequent phase, spermiogenesis, the spermatids undergo differentiation, each one eventually forming a sperm. The changes include formation of the acrosome or nuclear cap, the head, midpiece and tail (Fig. 3.4).

In the process a droplet of the spermatid cytoplasm is retained temporarily between the head and midpiece of the sperm and this is often seen in immature spermatozoa. The whole process of spermatogenesis takes approximately 60 days in the bull. Each sperm cell weighs approximately 2.5×10^{-11} g, half of which is contained in the head. The head is largely taken up by the nucleus, which contains the genetic material.

Spermatogenesis is essentially controlled by follicle stimulating hormone (FSH), which appears to act on the Sertoli cells. These in turn control the rate of spermatogenesis, although the mechanism for this is unclear. The presence of adequate concentrations of testosterone is also required. The Sertoli cells are also the source of inhibin, a polypeptide hormone which enters the systemic

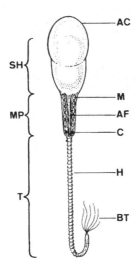

Fig. 3.4 Morphological structure of a sperm. SH, sperm head; MP, midpiece; T, tail; AC, acrosome; M, mitochondria; AF, axial filaments which begin in midpiece, extend through tail and emerge as a brush (BT) at tip of tail; C, ring centriole; H, helix which coils round surface.

circulation to selectively suppress FSH secretion by the pituitary gland. The hormonal relationships controlling testosterone production and spermatogenesis are illustrated in Fig. 3.5.

Hormone secretion in the male is pulsatile, as in the female. Each pulse of LH and FSH is followed by a pulse of testosterone (see Fig. 3.1). Testosterone in turn exerts a negative feedback effect, suppressing further pulses of LH secretion for a variable period of time.

Sperm transport in the male

After formation, spermatozoa are transported slowly by peristaltic muscle contractions, through the epididymis (Fig. 2.7) where they undergo further maturation. This occurs mainly in the epididymal caput (head) and corpus (body). Mature, fertile sperm are then stored in the cauda epididymis (tail) and in the proximal vas deferens. Normally about 30–35% of spermatozoa would be found in the caput and corpus, 50–55% in the cauda and 10–15% in the vas deferens, respectively. The frequency of ejaculation influences the transit time of sperm through the cauda epididymis but not through the caput and corpus. Average transit time through the caput and corpus is of the order of two or three days, and through the cauda, three to five days (Amann & Schanbacher, 1983).

The process of sperm maturation in the epididymis includes changes in morphology and metabolism and an increase in motility. These processes appear to

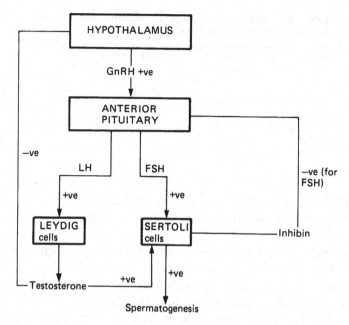

Fig. 3.5   Interrelationships between the testis, hypothalamus and pituitary gland in the control of male reproductive function.

be dependent on the presence of dihydrotestosterone, a derivative of testosterone, and possibly aldosterone, from the adrenal cortex.

Rate of sperm production

Within limits, the frequency of ejaculation does not affect the fertilizing capacity of sperm since the transit time through the epididymis does not vary greatly. The number of sperm in the cauda is maximal if the bull has not ejaculated for 7–10 days but is reduced by about 25% in bulls ejaculating on alternate days. If ejaculation is infrequent, the majority of unused sperm are voided during urination and few are reabsorbed. The rate of sperm production in normal adult males is fairly consistent within breeds and is correlated with testis size. Representative values for mature bulls of various breeds are shown in Table 3.1.

Composition of semen

The volume of semen produced in each ejaculate is highly variable both within and between bulls. It may vary from 1–2 ml in young bulls to up to 15 ml in older large bulls. However, the average volume is probably between 5 and 6 ml per ejaculate. Similarly, the sperm concentration can vary from zero in

Table 3.1 Sperm production in mature bulls. (From Amann & Schanbacher, 1983.)

Breed	Paired testes weight (g)	Daily sperm production	
		Per gram of tissue ($\times 10^6$)	Per bull ($\times 10^9$)
Hereford	650	10	5.9
Charolais	775	13	8.9
Holstein	725	12	7.5

azoospermic bulls up to 3000×10^6 per ml in exceptional bulls. As discussed above, the sperm concentration tends to decrease with a high frequency of ejaculation.

Although the testicle lobular tissue secretes a small proportion of the total seminal fluid, the accessory sex organs secrete the majority. Seminal fluid has a pH of about 6.5 and contains inorganic ions, fructose and other carbohydrates, citric, sialic and ascorbic acids, steroid hormones and a variety of other compounds. The seminal vesicles contribute the largest volume to the seminal fluid.

Semen quality

A number of parameters are used to assess the quality of semen. They include volume, sperm concentration, sperm motility, proportion of live sperm, proportion of abnormal sperm and a number of biochemical measurements and functional tests. There is a great deal of variation both between ejaculates and between bulls in all of these parameters and their relative importance in determining fertility has been open to debate (Watson, 1979).

Volume of semen may be important in relation to the number of semen doses that can be prepared from a single ejaculate. Density of spermatozoa is also of obvious importance in determining the number of semen doses and/or fertilizing capacity of the semen. The exhibition of progressive motility is important since it gives an approximate assessment of the viability of the semen. However, accurate determination of the ratio of live to dead sperm is carried out using differential staining techniques.

Sperm morphology

Blom (1983) categorized sperm defects in bulls and devised the spermiogram shown in Fig. 3.6. This lists and illustrates the most common sperm morphological defects that are seen in bull semen. Morphological examination of spermatozoa is accepted as a more meaningful technique of differentiating between semen of high and low fertilizing capacity.

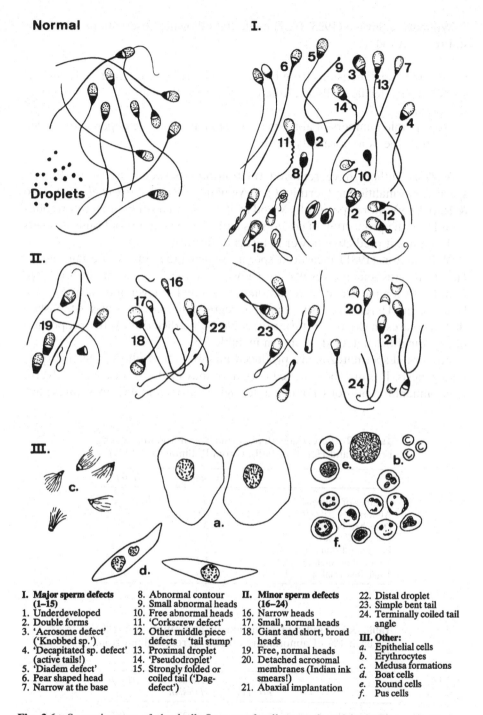

Normal

Droplets

I.

II.

III.

I. **Major sperm defects (1–15)**
1. Underdeveloped
2. Double forms
3. 'Acrosome defect' ('Knobbed sp.')
4. 'Decapitated sp. defect' (active tails!)
5. 'Diadem defect'
6. Pear shaped head
7. Narrow at the base
8. Abnormal contour
9. Small abnormal heads
10. Free abnormal heads
11. 'Corkscrew defect'
12. Other middle piece defects 'tail stump'
13. Proximal droplet
14. 'Pseudodroplet'
15. Strongly folded or coiled tail ('Dag-defect')

II. **Minor sperm defects (16–24)**
16. Narrow heads
17. Small, normal heads
18. Giant and short, broad heads
19. Free, normal heads
20. Detached acrosomal membranes (Indian ink smears!)
21. Abaxial implantation
22. Distal droplet
23. Simple bent tail
24. Terminally coiled tail angle

III. **Other:**
a. Epithelial cells
b. Erythrocytes
c. Medusa formations
d. Boat cells
e. Round cells
f. Pus cells

Fig. 3.6 Spermiogram of the bull. Survey of cell types found in bull semen. (From Blom, 1983.)

Williams & Savage (1925, 1927) made the following observations, which are still relevant today:

- Sperm head dimensions from bulls of good fertility are remarkably similar.
- No highly fertile bulls are found with more than about 17% abnormal sperm.
- Acceptable numbers of abnormal sperm in an ejaculate depend very much on the type of abnormality present.

Various authors have reported relationships between the proportion of sperm abnormalities and fertility (e.g., Aguilar, 1978; Salisbury *et al.*, 1978; Rao & Rao, 1979). More specifically Wood *et al.* (1986) in a study of Hereford bulls found that the proportion of coiled tails and of proximal protoplasmic droplets had significant predictive power in terms of fertility.

Willmington (1981) measured sperm abnormalities in 53 Friesian and 45 Hereford bulls and the results are shown in Table 3.2. The main difference found between the breeds was that there was a higher level of detached sperm heads in the Herefords. Using multiple regression analysis it was established that decreases in the non-return rate could be predicted from the proportion of abnormalities detected, as shown in Table 3.3.

Abnormal spermatozoa are produced mainly as a result of defective spermatogenesis. This may be genetic in origin or may be due to disease or adverse environmental conditions. For example, high environmental temperatures have

Table 3.2 Percentage of abnormal sperm found in young Friesian and Hereford bulls. (From Willmington, 1981.)

	Friesians	*Herefords*
Number of animals	53	45
Abnormal heads (%)	2.5	3.3
Detached heads (%)	2.5	5.7
Coiled tails (%)	1.6	1.9
Proximal droplets (%)	2.7	2.9
Minor abnormalities (%)	5.7	5.2
Total abnormal sperm (%)	14.9	19.1

Table 3.3 Predicted reduction in non-return rate (%) for each 1% of abnormality present. (From Willmington, 1981.)

	Young Friesian	*Adult Friesian*	*Hereford*
Abnormal heads	0.64	0.22	0.27
Detached heads	0.5	—	—
Coiled tails	0.77	—	—
Minor abnormalities	—	—	0.20

been reported to cause an increase in the proportion of sperm abnormalities (see review by Gwazdauskas *et al.*, 1980). Furthermore, bull fertility and semen quality are known to be seasonally variable (Parkinson, 1985). Functional tests include the measurement of hypo-osmotic swelling, sperm penetration into cervical mucus and in vitro fertilization tests.

Mating behaviour in the bull

As the onset of oestrus approaches in the female, she becomes attractive to the bull due to olfactory stimuli that are probably pheromonal. The bull approaches the oestrous cow and sniffs the perineal area. During this process, accessory secretions may drip from the prepuce. Mounting may be attempted several times before the cow will stand still. The act of copulation is very short, just a few seconds. The bull mounts, and the penis becomes erect, there may be a few exploratory movements of the penis, it is then inserted into the vagina (intromission), the ejaculatory thrust occurs, being followed immediately by withdrawal and dismounting.

Erection

The penis is composed of three cylinders of erectile tissue. These consist largely of sinuses, which during erection become engorged with blood rendering the organ turgid. In the farm species there is a relatively small quantity of erectile tissue so that there is little increase in size of the penis during erection. Most of the elongation is brought about by a straightening of the sigmoid flexure (Fig. 2.7).

Erection occurs following stimulation of the nerves of the parasympathetic branch of the autonomic nervous system which causes dilation of the arterial blood supply to the penis, thus increasing influx of blood. This also causes the contraction of the ischio-cavernosus (erector-penis) and bulbo-cavernosus muscles (Fig. 2.7), which prevent venous drainage from the penile tissue. The pressure of blood in the sinuses of the penis can reach ten times that of normal peripheral blood pressure. Full extension of the penis in bulls may be up to 55 cm (Seidel & Foote, 1969).

Ejaculation

The process of ejaculation occurs as a result of a wave of peristaltic contractions from the epididymis, along the vas deferens to the urethra. At the same time the walls of the accessory glands contract, forcing their secretions into the urethra. Ejaculation occurs on average approximately one second after contact of the penis and vulva. Full erection and ejaculation are almost simultaneous, with the ejaculatory thrust being accompanied by a slight twisting of the glans penis. Semen is deposited in the anterior vagina, just posterior to the external os of the cervix. There is some evidence that oxytocin release from the posterior pituitary gland may be involved in the ejaculatory process. After ejaculation, the penis is withdrawn into the prepuce by the action of the retractor penis muscle (Fig. 2.7).

Libido

Bull libido, or sex drive, is an important aspect of fertility, especially if the bull is used for natural service. There is a large genetic component to libido (Chenoweth, 1997) and it has been correlated with hormonal parameters such as oestrogen:testosterone ratios, which tend to be higher in low libido bulls (Henney *et al.*, 1990). However, Landaeta-Hernández *et al.* (2001) reported poor repeatability within bulls of results of tests of libido, service rate and reaction time to service, suggesting that mating behaviour is also under other influences, such as learning and/or environmental factors.

References

Aguilar, R.R. (1978) *Dissertation Abstracts*, **39**, 2031.

Amann, R.P. & Schanbacher, B.D. (1983) *Journal of Animal Science*, **57** (Suppl. 2), 382.

Blom, E. (1983) *Nordic Veterinary Medicine*, **35**, 105.

Chenoweth, P.J. (1997) *Veterinary Clinics of North America–Food Animal Practice* **13**, 331–344.

Fossland, R.G. & Schultz, A.B. (1961) *University of Nebraska Agriculture Experimental Station Research Bulletin*, **199**.

Gwazdauskas, F.C., Bame, J.A., Aalseth, D.L., Vinson, W.E., Saacke, R.G. & Marshall, C.E. (1980) *Proceedings of the 8th International Conference on AI Reproduction*, **13**.

Henney, S.R., Killian, G.J. & Deaver, D.R. (1990) *Journal of Animal Science*, **68**, 2784–2792.

Landaeta-Hernández, A.J., Chenoweth, P.J. & Berndtson, W.E. (2001) *Animal Reproduction Science*, **66**, 151–160.

Parkinson, T.J. (1985) *Veterinary Record*, **117**, 303.

Pelletier, S., Carrez-Camous, S. & Thiery, J.C. (1981) *Journal of Reproduction and Fertility* (Suppl. 30), 92.

Rao, T.L.N. & Rao, A.R. (1979) *Indian Veterinary Journal*, **56**, 33.

Rawlings, N.C., Fletcher, P.W., Henricks, D.M. & Hill, J.R. (1978) *Biology of Reproduction*, **19**, 1108.

Salisbury, G.W., VanDemark, N.L. & Lodge, J.R. (1978) *Physiology of Reproduction and Artificial Insemination of Cattle*. W.H. Freeman and Co., San Francisco.

Schams, D., Gombe, S., Schallenberger, E., Reinhardt, V. & Claus, R. (1978) *Journal of Reproduction and Fertility*, **54**, 145.

Schams, D., Schallenberger, E., Gombe, S. & Karg, H. (1981) *Journal of Reproduction and Fertility* (Suppl. 30), 103.

Seidel, G.E. & Foote, R.H. (1969) *Journal of Reproduction and Fertility*, **20**, 313.

Watson, P.F. (1979) *Oxford Reviews of Reproductive Biology*, **1**, 283.

Williams, W.W. & Savage, A.W.L. (1925) *Cornell Veterinarian*, **15**, 353.

Williams, W.W. & Savage, A.W.L. (1927) *Cornell Veterinarian*, **17**, 374.

Willmington, J.A. (1981) *Some investigations into the effect of sperm morphology on the fertility of bovine semen used for artificial insemination.* Paper presented to Association of Veterinary Teachers and Research Workers Annual Conference.

Wolf, F.R., Almquist, J.O. & Hale, E.B. (1965) *Journal of Animal Science*, **24**, 761.

Wood, P.D.P., Foulkes, J.A., Shaw, R.C. & Melrose, D.R. (1986) *Journal of Reproduction and Fertility*, **76**, 783.

Chapter 4
The Ovarian Cycle

The anatomical features of the female reproductive system were described in Chapter 2. Cellular division of oocytes begins early in fetal life. Division is arrested at the diplotene stage of the first meiotic division, only to resume at the onset of the oestrous cycle in follicles destined for ovulation. At birth, the ovaries of the female calf contain all the oocytes she will ever produce – from 200 000 up to about half a million. This is in contrast to the male in which sperm production is a continuous process during periods of sexual activity. Although the very young animal is sexually inactive and is unable to ovulate, it is apparent that some ovarian follicle development occurs even during the immediate postnatal period. From this early age waves of follicles begin to develop and migrate to the surface of the ovary. In the absence of stimulation by gonadotropic hormones these follicles fail to ovulate and become atretic.

Puberty in heifers

Puberty may be defined as the time at which oestrus first occurs, being accompanied by ovulation. The age of onset of puberty is clearly important since this could possibly prevent an animal's availability for breeding at the desired time (see Chapter 14). Timing of puberty is highly variable and, as with bulls, is dependent on a number of genetic and environmental factors, the most important of which are discussed below.

Factors affecting timing of puberty

Breed

Whilst there are few recent comparisons of breed type in the literature, dairy breeds appear to reach puberty earlier than beef breeds. The average ages and weights at which heifers of different types reached puberty are shown in Table 4.1 and, generally speaking, larger-type heifers (e.g., Simmental) were younger and heavier at puberty than smaller-type heifers (e.g., Angus) (Ferrell, 1982). Whilst breed and type may affect the age at puberty, it is clear that environmental influences also exert strong effects on prepubertal development.

Table 4.1 Age and weight of various breeds of heifers at puberty. (From Ferrell, 1982.)

Breed	Age at puberty (days)	Weight at puberty (kg)
Angus	410	309
Hereford	429	302
Red Poll	355	270
Brown Swiss	317	305
Charolais	388	355
Simmental	348	328

Nutrition, body weight and liveweight gain

It has been known for many years that nutritional status and the rate of liveweight gain are important determinants of the time of onset of puberty. In a study of the effect of different planes of nutrition, Ferrell (1982) showed that there was a negative relationship between age at puberty and the rate of liveweight gain, i.e., the faster-growing heifers reached puberty at a younger age. Under average conditions reproductive cycles would be expected to commence in Holstein/Friesian heifers at an average body weight of 250–270 kg. Heifers fed on very high planes of nutrition may achieve puberty as early as 5–6 months of age although this would be very costly in terms of feed. There is also evidence that the rearing of heifers at daily rates of liveweight gains of 1 kg and above may result in poor lactational performance subsequently, due to an inhibition of mammary growth (Sejrsen *et al.*, 1982). Under adequate conditions of nutritional management the onset of puberty in heifers is unlikely to be a limiting factor in the achievement of calving at two years of age as commonly practised in many countries. Nutritional influences on the onset of cycling are mediated by hormones such as insulin-like growth factors I and II (IGF-I and IGF-II), insulin and leptin. They are more likely to be limiting in lactating cows and their action is discussed in Chapter 7.

Season

There are many reports that season of birth may influence the onset of puberty in heifers; however, the evidence is often conflicting. A possible explanation of such inconsistencies is that exposure to different seasons during prepubertal development may also have an influence (Hansen, 1985). Photoperiod appears to be a major seasonal factor although temperature, particularly if extreme, may also be involved. Petitclerc *et al.* (1981) and Hansen *et al.* (1983) showed that supplemental lighting will reduce the age of attainment of puberty. The stimulatory effects of increased lighting appear to be equally effective at either high or low planes of nutrition.

Other influences

In addition to these seasonal effects on puberty, there has been one report of an influence of the phase of the moon on the time of oestrus (Roy *et al.*, 1980). The frequency of occurrence of first oestrous periods in 57 heifers showed four distinct peaks at approximately seven-day intervals and appeared to be related to the timing of the full moon. However, to our knowledge this work has never been confirmed or repeated.

The stimulatory effect of the presence of the male on the onset of puberty is well established in the gilt (see Hughes & Varley, 1980) and ewe (Dyrmundsson, 1981). Although there has been little research carried out on this aspect in cattle, one report suggests that a pheromonal compound present in bull urine can hasten the onset of puberty in heifers. Puberty occurred earlier when bull urine was placed directly in the vomeronasal organ than when water was placed there (Izard & Vandenbergh, 1982).

Roberson *et al.* (1987) penned heifers with or without exposure to mature teaser bulls from 9.5–15 months of age (152 days duration), but saw no effects on proportion of heifers reaching puberty. Conversely, in a later study conducted over a four-year period (Roberson *et al.*, 1991), heifers were exposed to or isolated from bulls from 11.5–14 months of age (76 days duration) and more of the heifers exposed to bulls were cyclic at initiation of breeding at 14 months of age. Mechanisms by which bulls or testosterone-treated cows reduce postpartum interval to oestrus are unknown.

Endocrine changes in prepubertal heifers

There have been few detailed studies of the hormonal control of the prepubertal period in heifers. It is known, however, that the release of pituitary gonadotrophins follicle stimulating hormone (FSH) and luteinizing hormone (LH) begins shortly after birth. In heifers that first ovulated at around nine months of age, plasma LH and FSH concentrations increased from birth to three months of age (Schams *et al.*, 1981) and then declined until about six months (Fig. 4.1). The values then increased gradually, peaking again at nine months. The occurrence of LH pulses could be detected at all ages but were of varying frequency. Injected oestradiol will result in LH release as early as three months of age (Schillo *et al.*, 1983). Elevated progesterone levels occurred for 8–12 days before the first oestrus, a phenomenon previously reported by Gonzalez-Padilla *et al.* (1975). An analogous pattern also occurs in progesterone profiles of some postpartum cows (see Chapter 7). These transient increases in progesterone in heifers were investigated by Berardinelli *et al.* (1979) who observed small luteal structures embedded within the ovary but not always observable on the ovarian surface. It is not clear whether these luteal structures are a product of a true ovulation.

At present the control of the transition to puberty in the heifer is not fully understood, but it should be clear from the foregoing that the various endocrine components appear to be functional in the prepubertal animal (Fig. 4.1). One

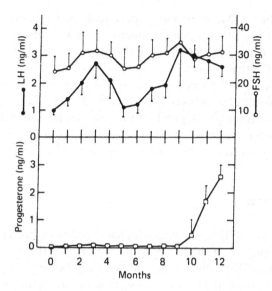

Fig. 4.1 Mean plasma LH, FSH and progesterone concentrations in four prepubertal heifers, from birth to 12 months of age. Note the decrease in LH concentrations between four and six months. (From Schams *et al.*, 1981.)

hypothesis as to the control of puberty at least in some species is the so-called gonadostat theory (see review by Foster & Ryan, 1981). Under this theory all components of the endocrine system become potentially functional shortly after birth. LH is released from the anterior pituitary gland and stimulates the production of oestradiol-17β from ovarian follicles. However, the hypothalamo-pituitary unit is excessively sensitive to the negative feedback effect of oestradiol and therefore LH secretion is inhibited. Eventually this excessive sensitivity is reduced, allowing gonadotrophin secretion to rise, thereby stimulating follicular development and eventual ovulation. The results of Schams *et al.* (1981) illustrated in Fig. 4.1 are clearly consistent with this theory, although this mechanism has not been conclusively demonstrated in the heifer.

Induction of puberty

Of the various attempts to induce puberty most have included trying to simulate the transient rise in progesterone that occurs prior to the first oestrus, by giving either progesterone implants or daily injections usually combined with either an oestrogen or pregnant mare serum gonadotrophin (PMSG) (Gonzalez-Padilla *et al.*, 1975; Rajamahendran *et al.*, 1982). The rationale for such treatment is that progesterone suppresses pituitary LH release, stimulating ovarian follicle development. Progesterone is also used to control the time of ovulation in the cyclic cow and to induce ovulation in the non-cyclic cow, and these topics are discussed later in Chapters 9 and 7, respectively. However, such treatments have only been consistently successful in animals considered to be already approaching puberty. More recent experiments have been carried out in younger heifers using either repeated injections or slow-release formulations of gonadotrophin releasing hormone (GnRH), but these also have so far failed to be consistently effective. Schoppee *et al.* (1995) used exogenous oestradiol-17β to induce the release of an LH surge within 12 hours of administration. They postulated that the effectiveness of the induced LH surge in inducing ovulation in prepubertal heifers might depend on the stage of follicular development at the time oestradiol-17β is injected. Regressing follicles or follicles that have not reached dominant status may be unresponsive to the LH surge.

The ovarian cycle

Since birth, waves of follicles (primary follicles) will have been developing and migrating to the surface of the ovary. In the absence of the factors required to mature and ovulate them, they cease to grow and begin to regress or degenerate, a process known as atresia. At puberty, the anatomical and hormonal conditions required for regular ovulation are established. The situation is analogous to that at the resumption of ovarian cycles after calving, which is discussed in detail in Chapter 7. Briefly, IGF-I and IGF-II will have stimulated the proliferation of small follicles and insulin will facilitate oestradiol production in follicles that could potentially ovulate, whilst the hypothalamic-pituitary axis becomes competent to produce the episodic release of LH necessary for follicle development and oocyte maturation and the LH peak necessary for ovulation.

The cow is a polyoestrous animal; therefore once oestrous cycles are established they continue indefinitely unless interrupted by pregnancy. This is in contrast to the ewe, for example, which is seasonally polyoestrous, i.e., it undergoes continuous oestrous cycles but only during certain seasons of the year. In the non-pregnant cow, ovulation occurs at approximately 21-day intervals. A short period before ovulation, the cow normally exhibits 'oestrous behaviour' or sexual receptivity (see Chapter 8), when she will attract and accept the attentions of a bull. Consequently there is a close relationship between ovarian and behavioural events, ensuring that the female is sexually receptive at the fertile period, i.e., about the time that ovulation takes place. The fact that she is not receptive at other times of the cycle is equally important, ensuring that the bull does not waste his resources when there is no chance of conception.

The oestrous cycle is classically divided into four phases:

- Oestrus, the period of sexual receptivity (day 0)
- Metoestrus, the postovulatory period (days 1–4)
- Dioestrus (days 5–18) when an active corpus luteum is present
- Pro-oestrus (days 18–20), the period just prior to oestrus.

However, these divisions are not particularly appropriate in the cow, as they are in other species, since the individual behavioural phases are rather indistinct. The cycle is better described in terms of ovarian function, as consisting of two components, the follicular phase (corresponding to pro-oestrus and oestrus) and the luteal phase (metoestrus and dioestrus). Behavioural oestrus occurs towards the end of the follicular phase.

The cycle is initiated by the release of gonadotrophin releasing hormone (GnRH) from the hypothalamus, which in turn causes the release of FSH from the anterior pituitary gland. This stimulates follicular growth. Of the cohort of primary follicles that has been recruited, and have developed to the antral stage (i.e., those containing a fluid-filled cavity), the most mature (the dominant follicle) responds to rising levels of FSH and becomes destined to ovulate (the pre-ovulatory follicle). The mechanisms regulating follicular development and the selection of the dominant follicle have been reviewed by Webb *et al.* (2003). The remaining antral follicles cease to grow and they also undergo atresia. This process is to an extent controlled by the production, from the dominant follicle, of inhibin, which acts at the local level in limiting the responsiveness of other follicles, and at the pituitary level by limiting the release of FSH. This mechanism ensures that most cows only ovulate one follicle during each cycle, since there are problems associated with attempting to carry more than one calf to term. About 1% of cows naturally produce twin calves as a result of two ovulations or of the division of the developing embryo to create identical twins. A small number of cows produce triplets and we are aware of two cases, one in Scotland and the other in Zimbabwe, in which cows have produced four healthy non-identical calves at one parturition. The use of exogenous FSH to overcome this inhibition and induce multiple ovulation is discussed in Chapter 13.

As the pre-ovulatory follicle develops, it continues to increase in size, eventually reaching a diameter of up to 2–2.5 cm. Insulin regulates the production of oestrogen by the theca interna and granulosa layers of the follicle. This oestrogen has three functions: (1) the initiation of oestrous behaviour, (2) the preparation of the reproductive tract for the processes associated with fertilization, and (3) the initiation of the ovulatory peak of LH.

(1) *Oestrous behaviour.* This typically lasts for between 6 and 30 hours with an average of about 7 hours. The duration of oestrus is dependent on several factors including age and season of the year and there also appears to be a diurnal pattern in that cows seem to show oestrus more frequently at night. The main sign of oestrus is that the cow will stand to be mounted by a bull, or by other cows in the herd. During oestrus the cow becomes increasingly restless and may bellow frequently. The vulva becomes swollen and the vaginal mucous membrane is deep red in colour. There is often a clear string of mucus hanging from the vulva. Visible oestrous changes are used to indicate the appropriate time for artificial insemination and are discussed in greater detail in Chapter 8.

(2) *Reproductive tract changes.* Oestrogen causes the retention of fluid in the cells making up the vagina, cervix, uterus and fallopian tubes. The whole

tract thus feels more turgid on palpation through the rectum. The resultant swelling tends to open up the passage through the cervix, allowing sperm to pass more freely and, fortuitously, facilitating the process of artificial insemination. The swelling also opens up the tubo-uterine junction for the passage of sperm and ova, and ensures that the infundibulum encapsulates the ovary, maximizing the chance that ova pass into the oviduct and are not lost into the body cavity. Oestrogen also increases blood flow to the reproductive tract and stimulates the production of mucus by the vagina, promoting the conditions for copulation. In the uterus, oestrogen facilitates the passage of larger cells, specifically white blood cells, into the lumen, increasing the resistance of the uterus to any infection which may be introduced at insemination. These secretions are expelled via the vulva, usually about two days after oestrus during so-called metoestrus bleeding.

(3)   *Initiation of LH release.* Increasing oestrogen levels from the pre-ovulatory follicle initiate a positive feedback response from the hypothalamus, so that a further GnRH release initiates the pre-ovulatory peak of LH.

Meanwhile, episodic releases of LH in a low amplitude, high frequency pattern [intervals of one per hour or more (Rahe *et al.*, 1980)], resulting in higher plasma hormone concentrations, will have contributed to the development of the follicle and the maturation of the oocyte within it (Fig. 4.2).

The pre-ovulatory LH surge itself consists of the summation of very rapid pulses of LH secretion. The surge (1) stimulates the process of ovulation, by activating an inflammatory reaction, which thins and ruptures the follicle wall (Espey, 1980) and (2) initiates luteinization of the granulosa and thecal cells of the follicle. The LH surge usually lasts from 7–8 hours and ovulation usually occurs from 24–32 hours after the beginning of the surge (Fig. 4.3).

At ovulation, the mature antral follicle ruptures, dispersing its content of follicular fluid in the abdominal cavity, and releasing the unfertilized ovum, still surrounded by cumulus cells. The ovum is collected by the fimbria of the oviduct and transported down the oviduct by a combination of cilial action and muscular contractions of the oviduct wall. Little is known about the mechanism of ovulation, but Bernard *et al.* (1984) reported visual observations of ovarian follicles over the ovulatory period using the technique of laparoscopy. About one hour before ovulation the follicle forms an 'apex', the point at which rupture eventually takes place. After ovulation there is a rapid collapse of the follicle wall.

As the pre-ovulatory follicle develops, the pre-ovulatory gonadotrophin surge acts on the oocyte, stimulating the resumption of meiosis, which had been suspended early in fetal life at the diplotene stage of the first meiotic division. The resumption of meiosis is characterized by breakdown of the germinal vesicle, chromosome condensation function of the first meiotic spindle, expulsion of the first polar body and arrest in the metaphase of the second meiotic division. These changes constitute oocyte maturation (Crozet, 1991).

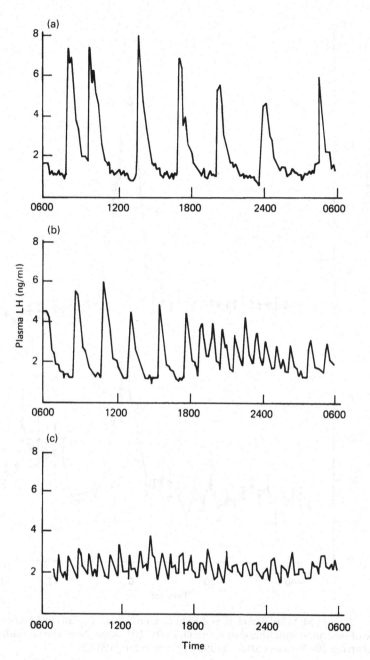

Fig. 4.2 Plasma LH concentrations in a cow on (a) day 10 (mid-luteal), (b) day 19 (follicular) and (c) day 3 (post-ovulatory) of the oestrous cycle. Note the high amplitude, low frequency pulses during the luteal phase and the increasing frequency and decreasing amplitude during the follicular phase. LH pulses are of low amplitude, high frequency during the post-ovulatory period. (From Rahe *et al.*, 1980.)

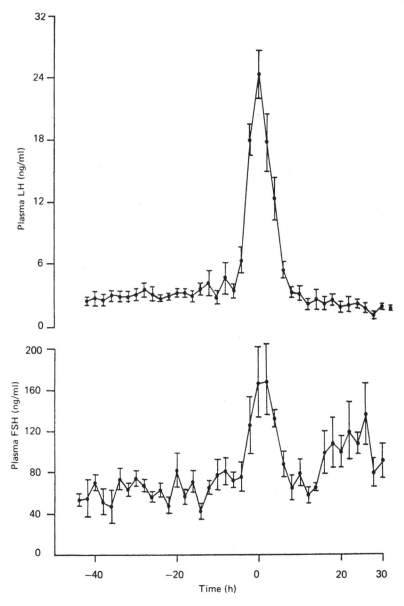

Fig. 4.3 Mean (± SEM) plasma LH and FSH concentrations (ng/ml) in 12 cows around the time of oestrus, standardized to the peak of the LH surge. Note the secondary FSH peak occurring 20–30 hours after the first. (From Peters, 1984.)

Expulsion of the first polar body occurs about 8–9 hours after the luteinizing hormone (LH) surge. Two cell divisions then occur quite rapidly, one just before ovulation and the other before fertilization. The first division is a meiotic division in which the chromosomal complement of the oocyte is reduced by half to 30. Instead of four cells being produced by these divisions only one is formed, plus a small 'polar body' at each division. These polar bodies are the 'other half' of the cell division but are deprived of most of their cytoplasm. The polar bodies invariably degenerate. Thus, as in the male, gamete production involves two meiotic divisions, but, by contrast, only one mature haploid gamete results from each primary cell.

Ovulation is considered to occur on day 1 of the cycle. However, as with the onset and termination of oestrous behaviour, the exact timing of ovulation is difficult to establish since continuous observation of the ovaries would be necessary. Most reports therefore have been based on discontinuous observations using techniques such as repeated rectal palpation or observation of the ovaries through a surgical incision in the abdominal wall. Consequently, reported values are quite variable. The literature is, however, unanimous that ovulation occurs some hours after oestrus. The average value reported is around 12–15 hours after the end of oestrus (see, for example, Schams *et al.*, 1977). The relative timing of the events associated with oestrus reported in that study is shown in Table 4.2.

In contrast, Bernard *et al.* (1984) suggested a very close relationship between the LH surge and ovulation, i.e., 27 hours from the beginning of the surge, and have used this to predict ovulation with considerable accuracy. It must be said here that these studies, now 20–30 years old, have not been repeated in detail in more modern genotypes of cattle.

After ovulation the cells remaining in the ruptured follicle proliferate and form the corpus luteum whose function then dominates the cycle from day 4 to about day 17. One of the functions of the LH surge is to cause differentiation of the follicular cells, including the switch from oestradiol to progesterone production (see review by Juengel & Niswender, 1999). Plasma progesterone concentrations begin to rise from about day 4 of the cycle, reaching a peak around day 8 and remaining high until day 17 (see Fig. 4.6). Pulsatile changes in progesterone concentrations occur during the luteal phase and these have been shown to be directly related to pulses of FSH from the anterior pituitary gland (Walters *et al.*, 1984). High amplitude, low frequency pulses of LH (approximately one every four hours) occur during the luteal phase, resulting in a low average plasma concentration (Rahe *et al.*, 1980). Although the LH pulse frequency is relatively low during the luteal phase, it nevertheless appears to be sufficient for the maintenance of luteal function. LH has been considered to be the main, if not the sole, luteotrophic hormone in the non-pregnant cow. Patterns of episodic LH release are shown in Fig. 4.2. As in other species,

Table 4.2 Relative timing of events at oestrus in the cow. (From Schams *et al.*, 1977.) All values are mean ± s.d.

	Time (h)	No. of observations
Duration of oestrus	16.9 ± 4.9	28
Interval, onset of oestrus to LH peak (max.)	6.4 ± 3.0	26
Duration of LH peak	7.4 ± 2.6	89
Interval, max. LH peak to ovulation	25.7 ± 6.9	75

episodes or pulses of LH secretion occur throughout the cycle, and their amplitude and frequency are dependent on the stage of the cycle. It is considered
that the pulsatile pattern of LH secretion is a consequence of pulsatile GnRH
secretion and this has been demonstrated in the female sheep (Clarke &
Cummins, 1982). In order to characterize in detail this type of hormone pattern,
it is necessary to take blood samples from animals at intervals of 5–15 minutes
for periods of 12–24 hours.

The primary role of high progesterone concentrations during the luteal
phase is to prepare the uterus for reception of the embryo that may have
resulted from fertilization of the ovum shed at ovulation. Progesterone also
exerts a negative feedback inhibition on GnRH and LH release, suppressing
further follicle maturation. Nevertheless, waves of follicles continue to grow
and regress, leading to transient rises in oestrogen levels (see review by Webb
et al., 1992). During each cycle, most cows undergo either two waves of follicle
growth approximately 10 days apart or three waves approximately 7 days apart
(see Fig. 4.4). It is likely that three wave cycles are more common in maiden
heifers.

In the non-pregnant cow, the corpus luteum begins to regress after about
day 17 – a process known as luteolysis. This is brought about by the influence

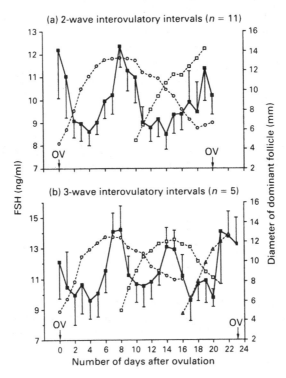

Fig. 4.4 Relationship between profiles of FSH (—■—) and growth of the dominant
follicle (---) for heifers with (a) two and (b) three follicular waves. OV, Ovulation. (After
Adams *et al.*, 1992.)

of uterine prostaglandin F2α (PGF$_{2\alpha}$), the release of which is initiated by oxytocin produced by the corpus luteum itself. Oxytocin is produced in the corpora lutea of both sheep and cows (Wathes & Swann, 1982) and plasma concentrations of oxytocin parallel those of progesterone during the oestrous cycle of the ewe. It is well known that exogenous oxytocin can induce luteolysis in the cow and that it has a physiological role in luteolysis by inducing the release of PGF$_{2\alpha}$. Specific oxytocin receptors are present on the outer membranes of endometrial cells in the uterus. Binding of luteal oxytocin to the receptor stimulates the conversion of arachidonic acid to PGF$_{2\alpha}$ within the endometrial cell. The concentration of oxytocin receptors is low during the early part of the cycle but increases as the cycle progresses, stimulated by oestradiol secretion from waves of follicle growth during the luteal phase.

This increase in oxytocin receptor concentration leads to the release of PGF$_{2\alpha}$ from the uterine endometrium via the uterine vein for transport to the ovary (see Fig. 4.5). From measurements of the relatively stable PGF$_{2\alpha}$ metabolite, 13, 14-dihydro, 15-keto PGF$_{2\alpha}$ (PGFM), it has been shown that PGF$_{2\alpha}$ is released from about day 15 of the cycle in a pulsatile manner and that secretion continues for several days or at least until progesterone concentrations are minimal (Kindahl *et al.*, 1981). The mechanism by which PGF$_{2\alpha}$ causes luteolysis has not been fully established, but the most likely possibility is that it inhibits LH activation of the adenyl cyclase system in the corpus luteum, preventing the production of progesterone by its large and small cells.

By approximately day 17 of the cycle, progesterone concentrations decrease to basal levels, initiating the events leading to the next oestrus and ovulation. As the corpus luteum begins to regress 3–4 days before oestrus, LH pulse

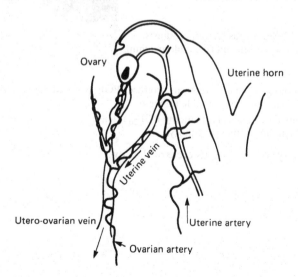

Fig. 4.5 Utero-ovarian vasculature in the sheep. PGF$_{2\alpha}$ is thought to leave the uterus via the uterine vein and is transferred to ovarian arterial blood by diffusion through the walls of the utero-ovarian artery. (Adapted from Baird, 1978.)

(1) The hypothalamus sends GnRH to the anterior pituitary, releasing FSH.

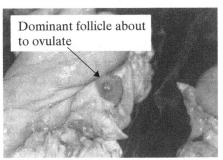

Dominant follicle about to ovulate

(2) The FSH causes the follicle to mature and the egg within it to develop.

(3) The developing follicle produces oestrogen which
    (a) induces oestrous behaviour;
    (b) acts on the reproductive tract causing oedema and ingress of white blood cells to combat infection;
    (c) feeds back to the hypothalamus inducing further GnRH release to the pituitary.

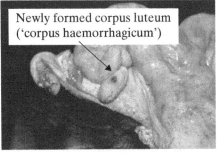

Newly formed corpus luteum ('corpus haemorrhagicum')

(4) This induces the release of LH.

(5) The LH causes ovulation–the release of the egg, which enters the oviduct (fallopian tube) to be fertilized and then continues to the uterus to implant and develop.

(6) The site of the follicle becomes the corpus luteum, which secretes progesterone, which
    (a) prepares the tract for implantation;
    (b) feeds back to the hypothalamus, preventing further ovulations.

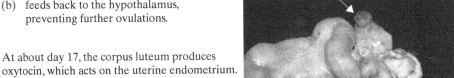

Mature corpus luteum

(7) At about day 17, the corpus luteum produces oxytocin, which acts on the uterine endometrium.

(8) (a) If there is no pregnancy, the uterus produces $PGF_{2\alpha}$, which destroys the corpus luteum and another cycle is able to begin.
    (b) If the animal becomes pregnant, the $PGF_{2\alpha}$ release is prevented, and progesterone levels remain high, supporting pregnancy.

Fig. 4.6 Summary of the oestrous cycle of the cow.

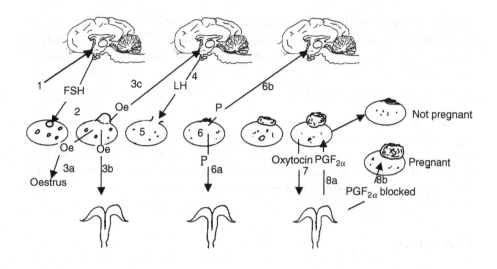

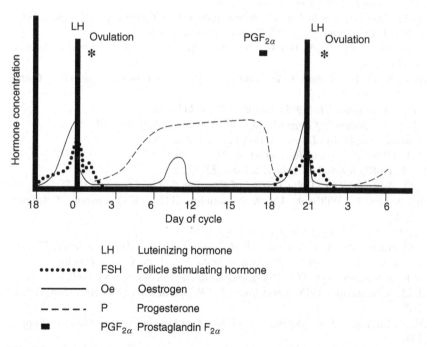

	LH	Luteinizing hormone
•••••••••	FSH	Follicle stimulating hormone
——	Oe	Oestrogen
– – – –	P	Progesterone
■	PGF$_{2\alpha}$	Prostaglandin F$_{2\alpha}$

Fig. 4.6 *Continued.*

frequency begins to rise. The fall in progesterone and rise in LH result in increasing oestradiol concentrations, which eventually 'triggers' the LH surge. As luteolysis proceeds, a new pre-ovulatory ovarian follicle begins to mature. If the animal becomes pregnant, the $PGF_{2\alpha}$ release is prevented, and progesterone levels remain high, supporting pregnancy, as described in detail in Chapter 5.

The sequence of events concerned with the oestrous cycle is summarized in Fig. 4.6. The typical cycle length is 21 days although there is considerable variation about this value. Most studies have shown that 80–90% of cows have a cycle length of between 17 and 25 days. There is some evidence that cycles are more regular and uniform in heifers than in adult cows.

References

Adams, G.P., Matteri, R.L., Kastalic, J.P., Ko, I.C.H. & Günther, O.J. (1992) *Journal of Reproduction and Fertility*, **94**(1), 185.

Baird, D.T. (1978) In *Control of Ovulation* (eds D.B. Crighton, N.B. Haynes, G.R. Foxcroft & G.E. Lamming), p. 217. Butterworths, London.

Berardinelli, J.G., Dailey, R.A., Butcher, R.L. & Inskeep, E.K. (1979) *Journal of Animal Science*, **49**, 1276.

Bernard, C., Valet, J.P., Beland, R. & Lambert, R.D. (1984) *Canadian Journal of Comparative Medicine*, **48**, 97.

Clarke, J.J. & Cummins, J.T. (1982) *Endocrinology*, **111**, 1737.

Crozet, N. (1991) *Journal of Reproduction and Fertility* (Suppl. 43), 235.

Dyrmundsson, O.R. (1981) *Livestock Production Science*, **8**, 55.

Espey, L.L. (1980) *Biology of Reproduction*, **22**, 73–106.

Ferrell, C.L. (1982) *Journal of Animal Science*, **55**, 1272.

Foster, D.L. & Ryan, K.D. (1981) *Journal of Reproduction and Fertility*, **30**, 75.

Gonzalez-Padilla, E., Wiltbank, J.N. & Niswender, G.D. (1975) *Journal of Animal Science*, **40**, 1091.

Hansen, P.J. (1985) *Livestock Production Science*, **12**, 309.

Hansen, P.J., Kamwanja, L.A. & Hauser, E.R. (1983) *Journal of Animal Science*, **57**, 985.

Hughes, P. & Varley, M. (1980) *Reproduction in the Pig*. Butterworths, London.

Izard, M.K. & Vandenbergh, J.G. (1982) *Journal of Animal Science*, **55**, 1160.

Juengel, J.L. & Niswender, G.D. (1999) *Journal of Reproduction and Fertility* (Suppl. 54), 193–205.

Kindahl, H., Lindell, J.O. & Edqvist, L.E. (1981) *Acta Veterinaria Scandinavica* (Suppl. 77), 143.

Peters, A.R. (1984) *Veterinary Record*, **115**, 164.

Petitclerc, D., Chaplin, L.T., Emergy, R.S. & Tucker, H.A. (1981) *Journal of Animal Science*, **57**, 892.

Rahe, C.M., Owens, R.E., Fleeger, J.L., Newton, H.J. & Harms, P.G. (1980) *Endocrinology*, **107**, 498.

Rajamahendran, R., Lague, P.C. & Baker, R.D. (1982) *Canadian Journal of Animal Science*, **62**, 759.

Roberson, M.S., Ansotegui, R.P., Berardinelli, J.G., Whitman, R.W. & McInerney, M.J. (1987) *Journal of Animal Science*, **64**, 1601.

Roberson, M.S., Wolfe, M.W., Stumpf, T.T., Werth, L.A., Cupp, A.S., Kojima, N., Wolfe, P.L., Kittok, R.J. & Kinder, J.E. (1991) *Journal of Animal Science*, **69**, 2092.

Roy, J.H.B., Gillies, C.M., Perfitt, M.W. & Stobo, I.J.F. (1980) *Animal Production*, **31**, 13.

Schams, D., Schallenberger, E., Hoffman, B. & Karg, H. (1977) *Acta Endocrinologica, Copenhagen*, **86**, 180.

Schams, D., Schallenberger, E., Gombe, S. & Karg, H. (1981) *Journal of Reproduction and Fertility* (Suppl. 30), 103.

Schillo, K.K., Dierschke, D.J. & Hauser, E.R. (1983) *Theriogenology*, **19**, 727.

Schoppee, P.D., Armstrong, J.D., Harvey, R.W., Washburn, S.P., Felix, A. & Campbell, R.M. (1995) *Journal of Animal Science*, **73**, 2071–2078.

Sejrsen, K., Huber, J.T., Tucker, H.A. & Akers, R.M. (1982) *Journal of Dairy Science*, **65**, 793.

Walters, D.L., Schams, D. & Schallenberger, E. (1984) *Journal of Reproduction and Fertility*, **71**, 479.

Wathes, D.C. & Swann, R. (1982) *Nature*, **297**, 225.

Webb, R., Gong, J.S., Law, A.S. & Rusbridge, S.M. (1992) *Journal of Reproduction and Fertility* (Suppl. 45), 141.

Webb, R., Nicholas, B., Gong, J.G., Campbell, B.K., Gutierrez, C.G., Garverick, H.A. & Armstrong, D.G. (2003) *Reproduction* (Suppl. 61), 1–20.

Chapter 5
Fertilization, Conception and Pregnancy

In order to achieve good reproductive efficiency it is necessary to maximize the chances of successful pregnancy at a given service or insemination. Therefore it is important to maximize both the fertilization rate and the conception rate and, furthermore, to be able to detect non-pregnant cows as early as possible so that appropriate action can be taken. The present chapter is concerned with the processes of fertilization and conception and the changes that occur during pregnancy.

Fertilization and conception

Much of the research carried out on fertilization has been conducted in species other than the cow; however, much of what follows refers to mammalian species in general.

At ovulation the ovum or egg is collected by the fundibular end of the oviduct or fallopian tube (see Fig. 2.11). It is transported down the oviduct towards the uterus possibly by a combination of cilial (hair-like) action and muscular contractions (see review by Overstreet, 1983). Transport through the oviduct appears to be under the control of ovarian steroid hormones since oestrogens reduce and progesterone increases the speed of passage of ova through the oviducts. Fertilization normally occurs in the ampulla section of the oviduct close to the junction with the isthmus (see Fig. 2.11; Hunter, 1980). In the cow, the ovum enters the uterus 4–5 days after ovulation.

Mammalian spermatozoa acquire motility, and part of their capacity to fertilize the ovum, during their passage through the epididymis. At the same time, they undergo changes in metabolic patterns, enzymatic activities, the ability to bind to zona pellucida surface, electrophoretic properties, and stabilization of some sperm structures. (Mújica *et al.*, 2003). However, before spermatozoa are able to fertilize the ovum, they have to undergo a further series of maturational changes in the female tract. These processes are known as capacitation and the acrosome reaction and are thought to require about six hours in the cow. This requirement for maturational changes is the main reason why it is preferable to inseminate cows several hours before ovulation (see Chapter 10). The precise changes involved in capacitation are not fully understood, but they involve enzymic and structural modifications to the acrosome and anterior part of the sperm head membrane. These include:

(1) an increase in membrane permeability to calcium
(2) modification of the membrane structure
(3) activation of the enzyme adenyl cyclase
(4) conversion of the protein proacrosin to acrosin.

The process of capacitation is stimulated when sperm enter the female reproductive tract. The acrosome reaction follows capacitation and involves the fusion of the sperm cell membrane and the acrosome and the formation of gaps through which the acrosome contents can diffuse. The acrosome reaction is necessary to allow penetration of the oocyte by the sperm. Capacitation and the acrosome reaction are very closely linked and therefore it is not always possible to distinguish between the two processes. The presence of ovarian follicular fluid and the cumulus oophorus have a stimulatory effect on the acrosome reaction but do not appear to be essential for it.

Spermatozoa transport

In the case of natural service, semen is deposited in the anterior vagina whereas with artificial insemination it is usual to place it just inside the uterus or in the anterior cervix. Spermatozoa ascend the female tract by both active and passive processes (Hunter, 1975). Active transport involves activity of the sperm tail or flagella, but clearly its interaction with epithelial surface secretions and cilia is also important. Propulsion of spermatozoa through the uterus appears to be quite rapid and the isthmus of the oviduct acts as a spermatozoa reservoir in many species. Recent observations using ultrasound techniques have demonstrated the capacity of the uterus to transport fluids to the vicinity of the oviduct in a matter of minutes (Brewin, personal communication; Sibley, personal communication), but not all observations have shown this consistently. Spermatozoa have been detected in the oviducts as little as two minutes after insemination (Van Demark & Moeller, 1951) although, again, others have failed to confirm this (Thibault *et al.*, 1975).

In other species it has been shown that after this rapid transport phase, the spermatozoa are cleared from the oviduct, possibly into the peritoneal cavity, and the oviducts remain free from spermatozoa until the pre-ovulatory period. This could explain the discrepancy between the observations described above. This rapid transport appears to be passive and due solely to uterine contractions of the female and has been demonstrated to occur even with dead spermatozoa. It is unlikely that such rapidly transported sperm would have any fertilizing function; most are found to be immotile (Overstreet, 1983).

On reaching the ovum, the sperm penetrates any remaining cumulus oophorus by the action of the enzyme hyaluronidase from the acrosome and comes into contact with the zona pellucida. The sperm nucleus possesses a cytoskeletal coat, the perinuclear theca (PT), which is removed from the sperm head at fertilization. The PT contains an oocyte-activating factor. This has not been characterized, but is thought to be responsible for triggering the signalling cascade of oocyte activation (Sutovsky, 2003). Mobility of the spermatozoa is also important in the process of sperm penetration.

Normally, only one sperm is able to pass through the zona, but when more enter, a process known as polyspermy, the resultant embryo is non-viable. Following fusion of sperm and egg, the contents of the cortical granules in the egg release into the perivitelline space (the cortical reaction), causing the zona pellucida to become refractory to sperm binding and penetration (the zona reaction). Sun (2003) discusses ways in which the cortical reaction may be mediated. Hunter *et al.* (1998) demonstrated that the ability of the zona pellucida to prevent the entry of another spermatozoon after fertilization persisted through to the blastocyst stage.

The fusion of the sperm and ovum cell membranes begins at the middle of the sperm head region. The sperm head becomes engulfed by the ova with the loss of the tall. The sperm's nuclear membrane disappears and the male chromatin comes into contact with the ova cytoplasm. Penetration by the fertilizing sperm (pronucleus) stimulates the resumption of the second meiotic division of the oocyte and the extrusion of the second polar body (see Chapter 4). Fertilization is completed with the fusion of the haploid male and female pronuclei, a process known as syngamy.

Pregnancy

Early development of the embryo

Gestation is often divided into three stages: (1) the ovum from 0–13 days, (2) the embryo from 14 days, when germ layers (see below) begin to form until 45 days, and (3) the fetus from 46 days until parturition. These divisions will be loosely used in the present text.

The ovum begins to divide mitotically, a process known as cleavage, immediately after fertilization is complete. Division continues so that a solid cluster of cells or blastomeres known as a morula (mulberry shape) is formed by five or six days. From about day 6 after fertilization, the ovum begins to hollow out to become a blastocyst. This consists of a single spherical layer of cells, the trophoblast, with a hollow centre, but also with a group of cells, the inner cell mass at one edge. The sequence of these events is illustrated in Fig. 5.1. The inner cell mass is destined to form the embryo, whilst the trophoblast provides it with nutrients.

At about day 8 the zona pellucida begins to fragment and the blastocyst 'hatches'. This is then followed by a period of blastocyst elongation. Development of the so-called germ layers begins from about the fourteenth day and characterizes the beginning of the embryo phase. The three germ layers

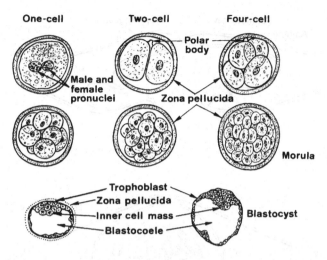

Fig. 5.1 Early development of the fertilized ovum to the blastocyst stage.

arise from the inner cell mass and are termed the ectoderm, mesoderm and
endoderm. The ectoderm gives rise to the external structures such as skin, hair,
hooves and mammary glands and also the nervous system. The heart, muscles
and bones are eventually formed from the mesoderm whereas the other internal organs are derived from the endoderm layer. By day 16, the embryo is sufficiently developed to signal its presence to the maternal system and prevent
the luteolysis that would have occurred if the cow had not been pregnant
(Chapter 4). This mechanism is described below under 'Hormonal changes
during pregnancy' on p. 63.

By day 45, formation of the primitive organs is complete and the fetal phase
is considered to have begun.

Formation of the extra-embryonic membranes

The embryo is able to exist for a short time by absorbing nutrients from its own
tissues and from the uterine fluids, but it ultimately becomes entirely dependent on its mother for sustenance. Therefore the embryo becomes attached to
the endometrium by means of its membranes, through which nutrients and
metabolites are transferred from mother to fetus and vice versa. The attachment process is known as implantation and may begin as early as day 20,
although definitive placentation does not occur until day 40–45 (see Fig. 5.4).

The yolk sac

This structure serves to transfer nutritive material from the uterus to the
embryo and is only of transitory importance in mammals. It is formed as an
outpouching of the developing gut (Fig. 5.2). It is separated from the uterine
wall only by the outer layer of the blastocyst and its blood vessels readily absorb

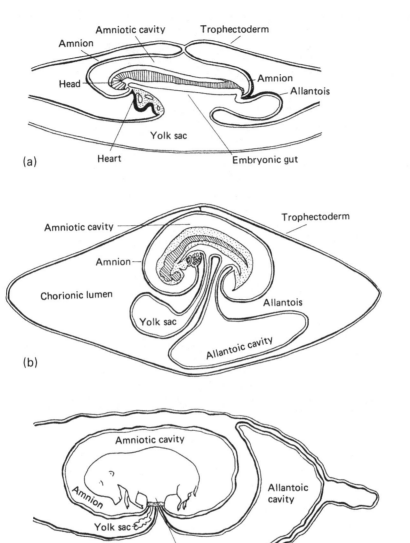

Fig. 5.2 Schematic illustrations of formation of the extra-embryonic membranes. (Redrawn from Patten, 1948.)

nutrients. The function of the yolk sac is eventually taken over by the allantois (see below).

The amnion

This membrane is composed of a layer of mesoderm and a layer of ectoderm, which grow up and over the embryo and eventually fuse to enclose it in a complete sac (see Fig. 5.2). The amnion is usually complete by day 18 and becomes filled with fluid, providing support and protection for the developing embryo. The amniotic sac is the so-called water bag that is often seen protruding from the vulva during first-stage labour (see Chapter 6).

The allantois

The allantois is formed as an outpouching of the developing hind gut. This grows outward, eventually coming into contact with the external layer of cells, the trophectoderm, formerly the trophoblast, to form the chorion or chorion + allantois (see Fig. 5.2). This membrane is usually well developed by day 23 and eventually surrounds the embryo, amnion and allantoic cavity, becoming densely vascularized, with the vessels branching away from the umbilical cord.

Placentation

The placenta is formed by intimate contact between the chorion and the endometrium. In ruminant species, the placenta is described as 'cotyledonary' since placental attachment occurs only in the discrete areas of the endometrial caruncles (see Fig. 2.9 and 2.10). Exchange of oxygen, carbon dioxide and nutrients between embryo and mother takes place solely through the cotyledons. By day 32 of pregnancy the allantois and trophectoderm almost fill the pregnant uterine horn and fragile cotyledonary attachment is also taking place there. A 12-week fetus and its associated membranes are shown in Fig. 5.3.

At the end of gestation the amniotic and allantoic cavities contain approximately 25 and 15 litres of fluids respectively.

Fetal development and other changes

Fetal growth is exponential throughout gestation, the rate increasing as pregnancy progresses. The average length of gestation is regarded typically as 280–285 days but is to some extent dependent on breed, particularly of the sire. For example, the effect of sire breed on the gestation period of Friesian cows is shown in Table 5.1. This shows that the continental beef bulls tend to produce longer gestation periods than Friesian and Hereford bulls.

Pregnancy appears to occur more commonly in the right uterine horn than in the left at a ratio of 60:40, with the corpus luteum typically being on the same side, reflecting the slightly more active right ovary as reported by several authors.

Approximately 1.4% of cattle births are twin births. Twins tend to be born prematurely (see Chapter 6) and to predispose to calving difficulties and retained placenta (Chapter 12). In cattle, as opposed to many other species, the fetal membranes of twin calves tend to fuse with each other, resulting in a direct vascular connection between the two fetuses. This means that if one fetus is lost, it is highly likely that both will be, and also predisposes to freemartinism,

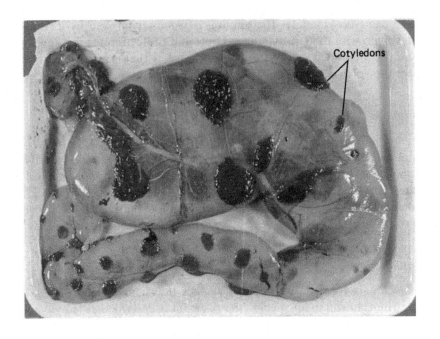

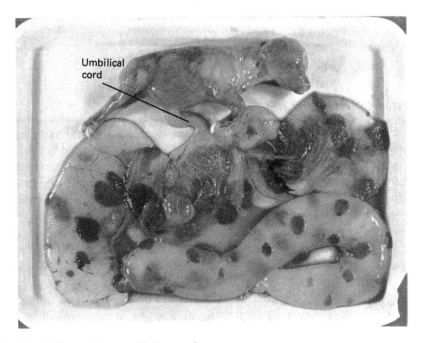

Fig. 5.3   A 12-week fetus with its membranes.

Table 5.1 The effect of sire breed on the gestation period of Friesian cows. (From Stables, 1980.)

Sire breed	Gestation (days)
British Friesian	281
Hereford	282
Charolais	284
Simmental	284
South Devon	285
Chianina	286
Blonde d'Aquitaine	287
Limousin	287

in which testosterone from a male calf interferes with the reproductive tract development of its female twin (see Chapter 12). Identical twins, derived from a single fertilized ova, or twins resulting from two ovulations on the same ovary are likely to begin development in the same uterine horn. The resulting over-crowding can increase the chance of loss, unless one of the calves can migrate to the contralateral horn.

A summary of the timescale of changes during pregnancy is shown in Fig. 5.4.

Hormonal changes during pregnancy

Oestrogen production

Ovarian follicle development continues during pregnancy as a result of low levels of gonadotrophin secretion. Both ovarian follicles and the embryopla-cental unit produce oestrogens. Changing ratios of this oestrogen and proges-terone can cause some cows to show oestrus during pregnancy (see Chapter 8), but this is not usually accompanied by ovulation. We are, however, aware of one case in which a cow was inseminated using Holstein semen and was re-inseminated with beef semen on showing oestrus three weeks later. She gave birth to twins – one Holstein and the other a beef breed.

In the pig, oestrone sulphate is produced from oestrogen of embryonic origin, which is then conjugated to sulphate in the endometrium. In the cow, plasma milk oestrone sulphate concentrations rise gradually during pregnancy and their measurement is a means of pregnancy diagnosis, as discussed in Chapter 11.

Progesterone and the antiluteolytic effect of pregnancy

Plasma and milk progesterone concentrations rise during the first few days of pregnancy in a similar manner to that occurring in the early luteal phase of the non-pregnant animal (Fig. 5.5). There are conflicting reports as to the time at

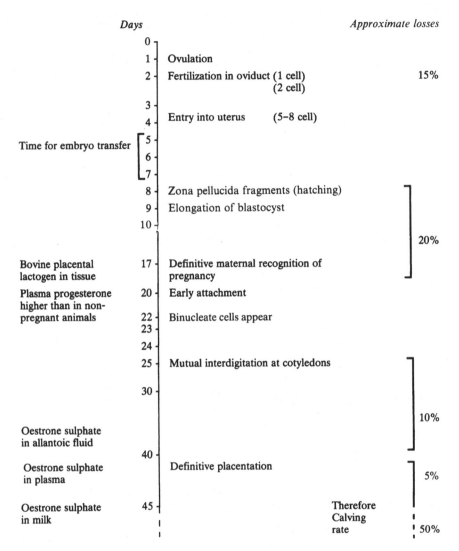

Fig. 5.4 Time scale of changes occurring during early pregnancy. (Reproduced courtesy of Prof. H. Dobson.)

which progesterone in pregnant cows begins to diverge from the non-pregnant pattern. Earlier work claimed that levels are different from as early as day 10 (Hansel, 1981), whereas others reported no differences until day 18 after insemination (Bulman & Lamming, 1978; see Fig. 5.5). More recently, it has been shown consistently that cows in which pregnancy fails tend to have lower progesterone concentrations in early pregnancy (Mann & Lamming, 1999; Mann *et al.*, 1999). It is apparent from these more recent studies that cows with lower progesterone levels as soon as day 5 after insemination are likely to have lower pregnancy rates, as shown by Starbuck *et al.* (2001) in a survey of 1228

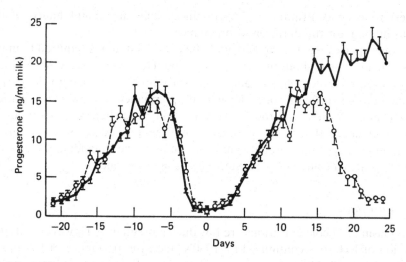

Fig. 5.5 Milk progesterone levels before and after first insemination (day 0) after calving in cows that did (●) or did not (○) conceive to that insemination. Each point is the mean ± SEM of 40 observations. (From Bulman & Lamming, 1978.)

Table 5.2 Relationship between milk progesterone concentration at day 5 after mating and pregnancy rate. (Adapted from Starbuck *et al.*, 2001.)

Milk progesterone on day 5 (ng/ml)	Approximate pregnancy rate (%)
<1	<10
1–2	30
2–3	40
>3	50

Holstein-Friesian dairy cows (Table 5.2). The significance of these and related findings to the diagnoses of pregnancy and the prevention of embryo/fetal loss is discussed in Chapters 11 and 12 respectively.

The increase in progesterone, through the mediation of progesterone receptors in the uterus, brings about alterations in the pattern of secretions into the uterus, thus preparing it to support the fertilized embryo (see review by Geisert *et al.*, 1992). It is generally considered that high progesterone levels are required for the maintenance of pregnancy. For this reason, the release of $PGF_{2\alpha}$ into the uterine veins, normally associated with luteolysis, is abolished in the pregnant animal. This is mediated by the conceptus itself, which, by day 16, has produced from its trophectoderm sufficient quantities of the protein interferon tau (IFNτ) to prevent the increase in oxytocin receptors that would otherwise be stimulated by oestradiol from ovarian follicles (Wathes & Lamming, 1995). Oxytocin from the corpus luteum thus fails to initiate the final stage of $PGF_{2\alpha}$ production and so, instead of declining from about day 17 or so, high progesterone concentrations are maintained, reflecting maintenance of the corpus luteum, for the duration of pregnancy.

In some species, e.g. the pig and goat, the corpus luteum is required to maintain pregnancy throughout the gestation period. However, in the cow, although the presence of the corpus luteum is necessary up to day 200 and the corpus luteum secretes progesterone throughout pregnancy, if cows are ovariectomized after 200 days, normal pregnancy will nevertheless be maintained. There is evidence that in the pregnant cow a major source of progesterone during pregnancy is the adrenal glands. In many species including the cow the placenta is also a source of progesterone during pregnancy.

Gonadotrophins

Mean plasma LH concentrations are low during pregnancy. However, pulsatile secretion of LH does continue. In a 1980's study the frequency of LH pulses decreased from 2.6/10 hours between days 50 and 60 to 1.2 pulses/10 hours between days 250 and 260 of pregnancy (Little *et al.*, 1982). Since LH is considered to be a major luteotrophic hormone in the non-pregnant cow (see Chapter 4), this low rate of LH release must be sufficient to maintain progesterone production at least during early pregnancy, unless other luteotrophic substances are involved. There is little information on the release of FSH during pregnancy, but it is logical to assume that it is secreted at relatively low levels. The placenta secretes a protein hormone, placental lactogen, which also has gonadotrophic properties (Bolander *et al.*, 1976).

A considerable research effort has been put into understanding the mechanisms governing the establishment and maintenance of pregnancy in farm animals. Of particular interest is the mechanism by which the early embryo is able to ensure its privileged position, protected from immunological attack, inside the uterus. This subject is of increasing importance to the livestock industry in view of the high rates of embryo loss, and it is likely that much research progress will be made in this field during the next few years.

References

Bolander, F.F., Ulberg, L.C. & Fellows, R.E. (1976) *Endocrinology*, **99**, 1273.

Bulman, D.C. & Lamming, G.E. (1978) *Journal of Reproduction and Fertility*, **54**, 447.

Geisert, R.D., Morgan, G.L., Short, E.C., Jr & Zavy, M.T. (1992) *Reproduction Fertility and Development*, **4**, 301–305.

Hansel, W. (1981) *Journal of Reproduction and Fertility* (Suppl. 30), 231.

Hunter, R.H. (1975) In *The Biology of Spermatozoa* (eds E.S.E. Hafez & C.F. Thibault), p. 145. Karger, Basel.

Hunter, R.H.F. (1980) *Physiology and Technology of Reproduction in Female Domestic Animals*. Academic Press, London.

Hunter, R.H., Vajta, G. & Hyttel, P. (1998) *Journal of Experimental Zoology*, **280**, 182–188.

Little, D.E., Rahe, C.H., Fleeger, J.L. & Harms, P.G. (1982) *Journal of Reproduction and Fertility*, **66**, 687.

Mann, G.E. & Lamming, G.E. (1999) *Reproduction in Domestic Animals*, **34**, 269–274.

Mann, G.E., Lamming, G.E., Robinson, R.S. & Wathes, D.C. (1999) *Journal of Reproduction and Fertility* (Suppl. 54), 317–328.

Mújica, A., Navarro-García, F., Hernández-González, E.O. & De Lourdes Juárez-Mosqueda, M. (2003) *Microscopy Research and Technique*, **61**, 76–87.

Overstreet, J.W. (1983) In *Mechanism and Control of Animal Fertilization* (ed J.F. Hartman), p. 499. Academic Press, New York.

Patten, B.M. (1948) *Embryology of the Pig*. McGraw Hill, London.

Stables, J.W. (1980) *The Bovine Practitioner*, **15**, 26.

Starbuck, G.R., Darwash, A.O., Mann, G.E. & Lamming, G.E. (2001) *British Society of Animal Science Occasional Publication*, **26**, 447–450.

Sun, Q.Y. (2003) *Microscopy Research and Technique*, **61**, 342–348.

Sutovsky, P., Manandhar, G., Wu, A. & Oko, R. (2003) *Microscopy Research and Technique*, **61**, 362–378.

Thibault, C., Gerard, M. & Heyman. V. (1975) In *The Biology of Spermatozoa* (eds E.S.E. Hafez & C.G. Thibault), p. 156. Karger, Basel.

Van Demark, N.L. & Moeller, A.N. (1951) *American Journal of Physiology*, **165**, 674.

Wathes, D.C. & Lamming, G.E. (1995) *Journal of Reproduction and Fertility* (Suppl. 49), 53–67.

Chapter 6
Parturition and Lactation

Parturition may be defined as the process of giving birth. This involves the preparation for and action of expulsion of the mature fetus from the security of the intrauterine environment into the harsher outside world. The process of reproduction in the cow is only successfully completed when a healthy neonatal calf is standing at its mother's side. Stillbirths and neonatal mortality may occur in up to 5% of calves. Therefore it is important that the complex process of parturition is understood in order that potential hazards may be predicted and possibly avoided. Parturition is accompanied by the onset of milk secretion or lactogenesis, so that the neonate is provided with an adequate supply of nutrients immediately after birth. The two processes are controlled by similar endocrine mechanisms and are closely synchronized. The present chapter describes normal parturition and its hormonal control together with problems that may arise, and, finally, there is a discussion of the process of lactation and its physiological control.

Hormonal changes at the end of gestation

The corpus luteum, placenta and adrenal gland all contribute to progesterone production in the pregnant cow. If the corpus luteum is removed during the last third of gestation the pregnancy will continue, although parturition may then be abnormal. It would appear therefore that the presence of the corpus luteum is necessary for the normal initiation of parturition. Plasma concentrations of progesterone begin to decrease gradually during the last 20 days of pregnancy and then fall more rapidly in the two or three days before parturition.

Parturition is an endocrine event, dependent upon the activation of the fetal hypothalamus–pituitary–adrenal (HPA) axis, as was demonstrated by the classical experiments of Liggins and coworkers in the early 1970s (e.g. Liggins *et al.*, 1973) in the sheep. It is assumed that similar mechanisms operate in cattle. For example, in the pregnant cow, plasma concentrations of corticosteroids rise about 15-fold during the last 20 days of gestation. This would appear to be important in the initiation of parturition, since the infusion of synthetic adrenocorticotrophic hormone (ACTH) into fetal calves also results in parturition within seven days. This could help to explain why twin calves tend to be born somewhat prematurely. The combined output of both sets of adrenal glands would result in threshold levels of corticoids being reached sooner.

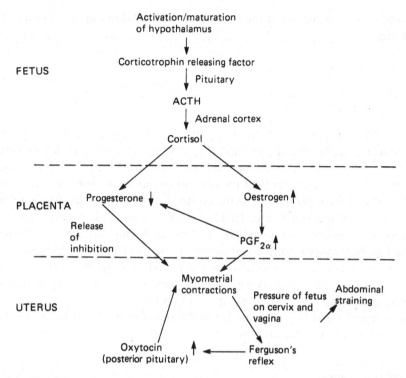

Fig. 6.1 Possible pathways for endocrine control of parturition.

In sheep and other ruminants, the increases in plasma concentrations of cortisol induces the activity of 17-hydroxylase and 1720 lyase in the placenta, increasing the biosynthesis of oestrogen relative to progesterone. This increase in ratio increases myometrial activity and culminates in labour and delivery. This process and its associated mechanisms were reviewed by Wood (1999); see also Purinton & Wood (2002).

Relaxin is a protein hormone secreted at least in part by the ovary and involved in the relaxation of the cervix and the fine control of myometrial activity before and during parturition. The putative sequence of endocrine events governing parturition in the cow is summarized in Fig. 6.1.

Parturition

Physical changes associated with parturition

Parturition or birth is classically considered to occur in three stages of labour:

- First stage – the preparatory stage, during which time the pelvic ligaments slacken and the cervix dilates.
- Second stage – expulsion of the fetus through the pelvic canal.

- Third stage – expulsion of the fetal membranes and initial involution of the uterus.

These will now be considered in more detail.

First-stage labour

First-stage labour consists of the preparation of the mother and fetus for the actual birth process. During this time regular contractions of the myometrium begin at a rate usually of 12–24 contractions per hour (Gillette & Holm, 1963). The cotyledonary attachments of the placenta begin to 'loosen' and the cervix shortens and dilates, partly due to the contractions, but also due to the breakdown of the collagenous tissue. There are often signs of discomfort, with the cow tending to bellow and possibly kick at the abdomen; she may also be restless and wander away from the rest of the group if at pasture or loose-housed. Also, the back is often arched and the tail raised. During this period the calf alters its disposition in that its forelimbs become extended in preparation for birth (compare calf disposition in Figs 11.11 and 6.2).

The length of first-stage labour is usually between 6 and 24 hours, tending to be shorter in older, parous cows.

Second-stage labour

This is characterized by the onset of regular contractions of the abdominal muscles compressing the abdominal contents. The myometrial contraction frequency increases up to about 48 per hour with 8–10 abdominal contractions occurring for each myometrial contraction. The cow will usually become recumbent during second-stage labour.

The myometrial contractions force the fetus backwards from the abdominal cavity into the pelvic cavity, which in turn causes the abdominal contractions

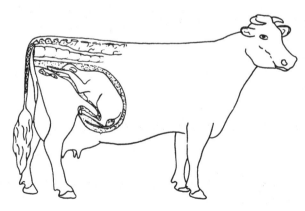

Fig. 6.2 Disposition of the calf immediately prior to birth. (Redrawn from Salisbury *et al.*, 1978.)

(straining). The pressure of the fetus against the cervix and anterior vagina stimulates the release of oxytocin from the posterior pituitary gland, which in turn stimulates further contractions of the myometrium. This mechanism is a typical neuroendocrine reflex arc and is known as Ferguson's reflex. The allantochorion is often ruptured quite early during second-stage labour with the escape of fluid through the vulva. As contractions proceed the amnion or water bag appears at the vulva and the calf's front feet are soon apparent inside. The amniotic sac may or may not rupture and, if it does, it provides lubrication to the calf's passage through the birth canal. After the calf's head has been expelled, abdominal contractions may cease for a short period before the rest of the body and lastly the hind limbs are expelled. The umbilical cord usually breaks spontaneously during expulsion of the fetus. Second-stage labour is usually completed in between 0.5 and 4 hours.

Third-stage labour

After expulsion of the fetus abdominal contractions cease; however, myometrial contractions continue, resulting in the separation and expulsion of the fetal membranes. This process may take up to 6 hours, but if longer than 24 hours it is likely to be due to a pathological cause.

After the fetal membranes have been expelled, myometrial contractions continue as well as the release of oxytocin and $PGF_{2\alpha}$. These factors result in an initial rapid rate of reduction in the size of the uterus. The pregnant horn is usually halved in diameter by about day 5 postpartum and halved in length by day 15. After this period the rate of involution is reduced, but in normal cows can be considered to be complete by day 30 postpartum (see Chapter 7).

Methods of induction of parturition

There has been periodic interest over the last two decades in the induction of parturition in cattle. However, the procedure has only really gained wide acceptance in New Zealand. This is mainly due to the fact that dairying in New Zealand is highly seasonal and lactation should coincide with maximum pasture availability. In the UK and other countries, the technique has not been popular because of the high prevalence of retained placenta, and reports of poor calf viability, reduced milk yield and reduced fertility. However, with the increased use of larger bulls in the UK it can be advantageous to advance the timing of parturition in order to minimize problems of dystocia due to fetal oversize. Also there are circumstances in which it is desirable to advance the time of calving to coincide with seasonal payments.

Corticosteroids

There is now a considerable body of information on the effects of corticosteroids on the pregnant cow. Parturition can be induced quite reliably from about day 255 of pregnancy onwards by a single injection of a synthetic gluco-corticoid such as dexamethasone, betamethasone or flumethasone. It is assumed that such therapy simulates the effect of the fetal adrenal cortex. A study was carried out (Peters & Poole, 1992) on the use of dexamethasone undecanoate to induce parturition in dairy cows in the UK. Cows were induced with 7.5 mg dexamethasone undecanoate (Dectan: Hoechst) either 14 or 5 days before term or left as untreated controls. The results are summarized in Table 6.1.

Dexamethasone treatment reduced gestation length by 10.8 and 4.3 days (significant reductions) when given 14 or 5 days respectively before the expected date of calving. Cows induced 5 days early calved sooner after injection (range 22–71 hours) than those induced 14 days early (range 40–190 hours). Induction of calving 14 days early resulted in a significant decrease in calf liveweight of 3.2 kg at one day of age. However, there was no significant difference in calf liveweights of cows induced 5 days early and their controls.

There were no significant differences in calving difficulty between induced and control cows. However, cows induced 14 days early tended to pose more difficulty in calving. These difficulties appear to have been related mainly to inadequate pelvic dilatation at the induced parturition. Dexamethasone treatment caused a significant increase in the time that the placenta was retained in both induced groups, although this was longer in the cows treated 14 days early (mean 3.5 days) than those treated 5 days early (2.5 days). Of the 17 cows induced 14 days early, 14 retained the placenta for 4 days whereas only 1/17 control cows retained the placenta for more than 12 hours. In the group induced 5 days early the problem was less marked, with 5/13 cows retaining the placenta for 4 days. The additional veterinary cost (excluding dexamethasone treatment) for cows induced 14 days early was £14.50 per cow and the cost differential for those induced 5 days early was £1 per cow. Calf survival over all treatment

Table 6.1   Effects of induction of parturition 14 days before and 5 days before term.

	Group A (induced 14 days)	Group B (control)	Group C (induced 5 days)	Group D (control)
Number in group	17	17	13	13
Gestation (days)	271.4	282.2	279.7	284.0
Liveweight after calving (kg)	518	505	605	574
Calf liveweight (kg)	37.4	40.6	44.0	42.2
Calving difficulty[a]	2.53	1.71	1.92	1.85
Placenta retained (days)	3.50	0.59	2.04	0.62
Calving to first service (days)	78.5	76.7	61.1	65.6
Calving to last service (days)	91.4	93.8	61.4	82.2
Total services	1.57	1.76	1.22	1.50
Pregnancy[b]	0.57	0.88	0.56	0.70
Milk yield in 100 days (kg)	2126	2279	2408	2565

[a] Based on scores of 1 to 5 where 1 = easy and 5 = very difficult.
[b] Where 1 = pregnant and 0 = not pregnant.

groups was 95%, with only three calves dying at birth and which were unrelated to any treatment group. There was no difference in subsequent calving to first service intervals between treated and control cows. Retained placenta possibly leading to endometritis was clearly associated with subsequent subfertility, particularly in the 14-day group. However, induction did not significantly affect either milk yield or quality.

Königsson *et al.* (2001) showed that cortisol profiles at parturition might be altered after induction of parturition with dexamethasone, leading in turn to retained fetal membranes. Induction of parturition using corticosteroids is now an essential part of management in many New Zealand dairy herds and considerable experience of the technique has been gained. Both short- and long-acting formulations have been used. Short-acting formulations, generally in the form of a soluble ester of the steroid, usually result in parturition 2–3 days later. Although the calves are usually viable, this method has been associated with a high rate of retention of the fetal membranes. The use of longer-acting corticosteroid formulations, for example a concentrated suspension of 'betamethasone alcohol' (MacDiarmid, 1979), resulted in a more protracted response, up to two weeks in some cases, and a high incidence of calf mortality.

In conclusion, parturition can be induced with dexamethasone undecanoate as early as 14 days prepartum with no adverse effects on calf viability or milk yield. However, an increased incidence of retained placenta may lead to increased veterinary costs and subfertility which may or may not be acceptable depending on the indications for induction. Induction nearer the time of parturition is unlikely to be associated with adverse side effects.

Prostaglandins

Prostaglandins, both $PGF_{2\alpha}$ and synthetic analogues, may be used to induce parturition in cows, although treatment before day 270 of gestation is not recommended. Parturition usually occurs between one and eight days after injection but at an average of three days. There is likely to be a higher incidence of calving difficulty, stillbirth and retained placenta, as reported, e.g., by Kornmatitsuk *et al.* (2002) who were also concerned with fetal well-being.

A study under UK conditions (Murray *et al.*, 1984) used a treatment regimen whereby cows were injected with 20 mg dexamethasone and those that had not calved 10 days later received an injection of 0.5 mg cloprostenol (an analogue of $PGF_{2\alpha}$. Although there was a high incidence of retained placenta, this did not affect subsequent reproductive performance. It was concluded that provided management was organized adequately to supervise parturition and take care of the neonates, then this procedure could be carried out to advantage.

A characteristic of early studies on the pharmacological induction of parturition was the high rate of calf mortality and post-calving problems, particularly retained placenta. An important determinant of the incidence of retained placenta appears to be the oestrogen status of the cow at the time of induction. As discussed above, oestrogen concentrations rise during late pregnancy, hence the oestrogen status may simply be a reflection of the proximity of term or 'readiness to calve'. From an exhaustive review of the available literature, First (1979) concluded that if induction is carried out when oestrogen levels are elevated, both glucocorticoids and prostaglandins are effective. However, glucocorticoids were the most appropriate treatment if induction was to be attempted earlier. The earlier that interference is attempted the higher the probability of calf mortality, retained placenta and other related problems.

Delay of parturition

It is now possible to delay parturition for several hours with pharmacological treatments. This is usually carried out so that supervision for calving can be more conveniently and readily available. Injection of the potent adrenergic drug clenbuterol inhibits myometrial contractions, thus slowing down the first stage of labour. However, if treatment is started after second-stage labour has already commenced, it would have little effect.

Lactation

Since a supply of milk is required for the neonate shortly after parturition, it is fairly logical that mammary development (mammogenesis) and the onset of milk secretion (lactogenesis) are under the control of similar hormones to those involved in the control of pregnancy and parturition.

The cow has four separate mammary glands and the same number of teats. Supernumerary teats are often present at birth, but they are usually removed early in life. The udder is suspended from the inguinal area by a system of ligaments which attach to the tendons of the muscles of the abdominal wall and inside thigh.

Structure of the mammary gland

Milk is synthesized in specialized epithelial secretory cells from substances absorbed from the blood. The basic secretory unit is the alveolus, a spherical structure consisting of a group of secretory cells surrounding a central cavity or lumen (see Fig. 6.3). The lumen is connected by a series of ducts of increasing size to the cisterna or lactiferous sinus from which milk is released via the teat. Each alveolus is surrounded by specialized contractile cells – the myoepithelial or basket cells (see Fig. 6.3). These cells contract under the influence of oxytocin from the posterior pituitary gland, expressing milk from the alveolar lumen into the duct system. Groups of alveoli, known as lobules, are separated from each other by connective tissue.

At birth there is little mammary development, with only the presence of teats, connective tissue and a few short ducts. There is an absence of the lobulo-alveolar system, with the space between the connective tissue occupied by fat

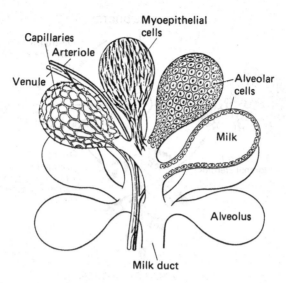

Fig. 6.3   Alveolar structure in the mammary gland. (Redrawn from Cowie, 1984.)

cells. Although further differentiation begins at puberty in many species, in the bovine it is only during pregnancy that marked development of the duct and lobulo-alveolar systems begins.

Control of mammary development

Much of the experimental work to elucidate the hormonal mechanisms of lactation has been carried out in laboratory animals, particularly rats, since it has involved complex techniques including surgical removal of endocrine glands coupled with hormonal replacement therapy. Hence there is a lack of direct experimental evidence concerning these events in the cow and therefore the following discussion extrapolates liberally from other species. A summary of the endocrine control of mammary development and the onset of lactation is shown in Fig. 6.4.

The endocrine glands involved in mammary development and lactogenesis are the anterior pituitary, ovary and adrenal gland. High concentrations of growth hormone, oestrogens and cortisol are necessary for ductal growth, whilst growth hormone, prolactin, oestradiol, progesterone and cortisol are required for maximal lobulo-alveolar growth. Lactogenesis, defined as the onset of copious milk secretion, is brought about by the hormonal changes occurring at the end of pregnancy and at parturition. The fall in progesterone concentrations at parturition appears to be the trigger for the onset of lactation.

Lactation can be induced in non-lactating heifers or cows by repeated injections of oestrogens and progesterone. This is not common practice in the UK but has wider appeal in other countries, such as New Zealand.

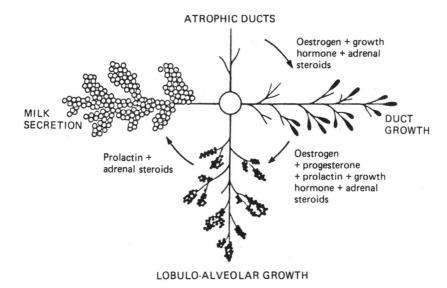

Fig. 6.4 Hormones and mammary development. (Redrawn from Cowie, 1984.)

Milk let-down

The milking or suckling stimulus is associated with the release of oxytocin from the posterior pituitary gland. Oxytocin stimulates contraction of the myo-epithelial or basket cells, expressing milk from the alveoli into the duct system (see Fig. 6.3). Expression of milk through the teat orifice is a passive process brought about by the sucking action of the calf or milk machine.

The composition of milk

Since milk is the sole source of food supply for the neonatal calf, it is natural that it should contain all the necessary nutrients to sustain the calf during the first days of life. Milk consists of two liquid phases, an aqueous and a fat phase, and a number of constituents are present in each. Lactose, minerals particularly calcium, phosphorus and magnesium and vitamins are present in the aqueous phase in solution while proteins are present in colloidal suspension. The lipid or fat phase contains vitamins and other fat-soluble components.

Lactose is the major milk sugar and is a disaccharide consisting of one glucose and one galactose moiety. Lactose provides twice the energy value per molecule of glucose and hence is a most efficient calorogenic substance. Milk proteins may be classified either as caseins or as whey proteins. Caseins are phosphoproteins which precipitate in acid conditions (pH 4.6) or under the influence of the enzyme renin. Caseins are specific to milk and serve as a supply of essential amino acids for protein synthesis in the young animal. Whey proteins do not precipitate at acid pH and consist of two types, the albumens and

Table 6.2 Average composition of bovine milk. (From Jenness & Sloan, 1970.)

	Composition (g/100 ml)
Total solids	12.7
Fat	3.7
Casein	2.8
Whey protein	0.6
Lactose	4.8

globulins. The globulins are largely the immunoglobulins, which confer passive protection against infections in the neonate. They are perhaps one of the most important components of milk from the point of view of neonatal calf survival. They are antibody proteins present in the dam's serum, which have been formed in response to exposure to microbial antigens and they thus confer protection to the calf against disease. Cows' milk has a high immunoglobulin content for only the first few days after calving (colostrum) and the calf's gastric mucosa is capable of absorbing the protein molecules for only the first 36 hours of life.

There are two main albumens in bovine milk, namely α-lactalbumen and β-lactagiobulin. α-lactalbumen is a specific milk protein and is identical to the so-called B protein, a portion of the enzyme, lactose synthetase, which catalyses the synthesis of lactose (see Mepham, 1976). β-lactaglobulin is misnamed and is, in fact, an albumen protein and is specific to the milk of cloven-hoofed species.

Milk fat is composed largely of triglycerides. These are derivatives of glycerol to which three fatty acid residues are linked. In contrast to other species, the milk of ruminants has a high proportion of short-chain (less than 10 carbon) fatty acids. Quantitative aspects of some milk constituents are shown in Table 6.2.

Maintenance of lactation (galactopoiesis)

Once established, milk secretion is usually maintained for approximately 300 days in the cow. The typical pattern of milk production is illustrated in Fig. 6.5 and demonstrates a rapid rise to peak production in the first 4–6 weeks, followed by a gradual decline over the next 8–9 months. Milk yield and composition are largely determined genetically (see Chapter 15); however, they can be manipulated to a limited extent by judicious control of feeding levels, particularly those of protein and energy (for reviews see BSAS, 1995).

Growth hormone from the anterior pituitary gland appears to be one of the main hormonal factors limiting milk yield and there is current interest in increasing yields using injections of growth hormone derived from recombinant DNA techniques.

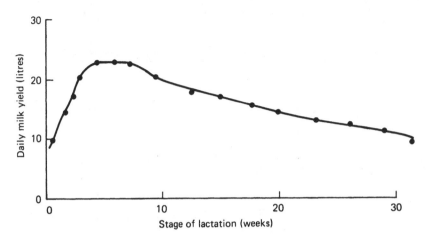

Fig. 6.5 Typical lactation curve of a dairy cow.

Cows are usually allowed to 'dry off' for the two months preceding parturition to allow regeneration of mammary tissue, thus ensuring maximum yield in the next lactation.

References

BSAS (1995) *Breeding and feeding the High Genetic Merit Dairy Cow.* BSAS Occasional Publication No. 19. Nottingham University Press.

Cowie, A.T. (1984) In *Hormonal Control of Reproduction* (eds C.R. Austin & R.V. short), 2nd edn, pp. 201, 211. Cambridge University Press, Cambridge.

First, N.L. (1979) In *Beltsville Symposia in Agricultural Research 3, Animal Reproduction* (eds H.W. Hawk, C.A. Kiddy & H.C. Cecil), p. 215. Alleheld-Osmun, Montclair, New Jersey.

Gillette, D.O. & Holm, L. (1963) *American Journal of Physiology,* **204**, 115.

Jenness, R. & Sloan, R.E. (1970) *Dairy Science Abstracts,* **32**, 599.

Königsson, K., Kask, K., Gustafsson, H., Kindahl, H. & Parvizi, N. (2001) *Acta Veterinaria Scandinavica,* **42**, 151–159.

Kornmatitsuk, B., Veronesi, M.C., Madej, A., Dahl, E., Ropstad, E., Beckers, J.F., Forsberg, M., Gustafsson, H. & Kindahl, H. (2002) *Animal Reproduction Science,* **72**, 153–164.

Liggins, G.C., Fairclough, R.I., Grieves, S.A., Tindall, J.Z. & Knox, B.S. (1973) *Recent Progress in Hormone Research,* **29**, 111.

Macdiarmid. S.C. (1979) *New Zealand Veterinary Journal,* **28**, 61.

Mepham, B. (1976). *The Secretion of Milk.* Edward Arnold, London.

Murray, R., Nutter, W.T., Wilman, S. & Harker, D.B. (1984) *Veterinary Record,* **115**, 296.

Peters, A.R. & Poole, D.A. (1992) *Veterinary Record,* **131**, 576.

Purinton, S.C. & Wood, C.E. (2002) *Journal of Physiology,* **544**, 919–929.

Salisbury, G.W., Vandemark, N.L. & Lodge, J.R. (1978) *Physiology of Reproduction and Artificial Insemination of Cattle.* W.H. Freeman, San Francisco.

Wood, C.E. (1999) *Journal of Reproduction and Fertility* (Suppl 54), 115–126.

Chapter 7
The Postpartum Period

The importance of the calving interval in determining reproductive performance was discussed in Chapter 1. The present chapter is concerned with the re-establishment of ovarian cycles after calving. This is an important component of the calving interval. Parturition is followed by a period of ovarian inactivity and sexual quiescence before reproductive cycles recommence. This is a possible natural mechanism for reducing the chance of reconception before the recently born calf has been weaned. The length of this interval is variable and can be affected by such factors as milk yield, suckling, nutritional status, inheritance and season. The relationship between the time taken to resume ovarian cycles (the acyclic period) and other reproductive parameters is illustrated in Fig. 1.1.

There is a transient increase in FSH 2–3 days after parturition followed by the re-establishment of waves of follicular growth. Normally, one follicle from each wave achieves dominance, as described in Chapter 2, the first dominant follicle being present by about day 10 postpartum (Roche & Diskin, 2001). It is by no means certain that this will initiate ovarian cycles, since a number of other conditions need to be met before a dominant follicle will ovulate:

- LH pulse frequency. This has been shown to be higher in cows that ovulate their first dominant follicle (Beam & Butler, 1999), suggesting that a threshold frequency is necessary to induce final follicle maturation and/or produce the ovulatory peak. Pulse rate is lower in cows that are still in negative energy balance, those that produce more milk and those with hypoglycaemia (Butler, 2001). Data from sheep indicate that exogenous IGF-I increases LH release (Adam *et al.*, 2000) and that circulating IGF-I may alter the sensitivity of the pituitary to LHRH and to oestradiol feedback (Snyder *et al.*, 1999), suggesting that IGF-I is the mediator for metabolic influences on LH release.
- Oestradiol secretion. A dominant follicle needs to produce sufficient oestradiol to trigger an LH surge and ovulation. Our own studies in beef cows have shown that the pituitary gland is able to release a normal pre-ovulatory surge of LH in response to exogenous oestradiol by day 14 postpartum.
- Insulin-like growth factors I and II (IGF-I and IGF-II). Systemic IGF-I, in addition to its effect on LH release, acts with locally produced IGF-II to encourage proliferation of smaller follicles in particular. IGF also enhances ovarian oestradiol and progesterone production.

- Insulin. The effects of insulin overlap to an extent with those of IGF-I, but insulin has a specific effect in stimulating oestradiol production by the follicle (Spicer & Echternkamp, 1995).
- Leptin. Decreased levels of this 16-kDa protein, produced in the fatty tissues, have been linked to delayed resumption of cyclicity (Kadokawa *et al.*, 2000; see also Chapter 12) and it is thought to be a further metabolic signal linking metabolism to reproductive performance. At the cellular level, leptin appears to inhibit the action of insulin on steroidogenesis and the stimulation of androgen production by LH (Armstrong *et al.*, 2003).

For reviews of these effects, see Armstrong *et al.* (2003), Diskin *et al.* (2003) and Wathes *et al.* (2003). Once a follicle has ovulated and provided that the requisite conditions are maintained, the cow resumes ovarian cycles, as described in Chapter 4.

Progesterone as an indicator of ovarian function

As blood plasma progesterone concentration directly reflects the activity of the corpus luteum, this is a precise indicator of ovarian function and has been used to monitor pregnancy, oestrous cycles and postpartum ovarian activity. Progesterone concentrations in milk closely follow those in plasma, the levels in whole milk being two or three times higher. As progesterone is highly soluble in fat, it diffuses preferentially into the milk fat.

Assay of progesterone in milk has two advantages over that of plasma: milk is easier to obtain and the assay procedure is simpler. This technique is used commercially as a method of early pregnancy diagnosis (see Chapter 11), as well as an experimental technique to monitor ovarian function (e.g. Lamming *et al.*, 1998). Progesterone may be measured in whole milk or in milk fat, and although each technique gives different values (see Bulman, 1979) the overall interpretation is similar. Traditionally, the addition of charcoal followed by centrifugation and decanting has been used to separate antibody-bound from antibody-unbound progesterone. Simpler methods are now available, such as magnetic separation available in kits from Amersham PLC and solid phase assays in which the antibody is bound to the plastic tubes used in the assay. After incubation and decanting, bound progesterone remains in the original tube for counting. One such kit, utilizing iodine 125 to label the progesterone, is produced and supplied by the International Atomic Energy Agency. Enzymatic (ELISA) assays normally rely on colour intensity as an indicator of progesterone levels. They obviate the need for handling radioactivity and for expensive gamma or beta radiation counters and are therefore more convenient for on-farm use. Milk progesterone profiles constructed from measurements in samples taken twice or thrice weekly from each animal have been used to monitor ovarian activity in postpartum dairy cows and suckling beef cows.

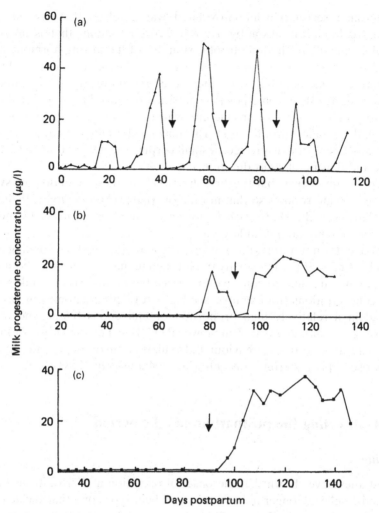

Fig. 7.1 Milk progesterone profiles of three postpartum cows. Note the short acyclic period for cow (a) and small transient rise in milk progesterone concentrations before onset of normal cycles. Cow (b) was acyclic for approximately 78 days. Arrows indicate days of oestrus. Cow (c) was served by a bull on day 90 postpartum before any rise in milk progesterone concentrations and became pregnant to this service, as shown by continuous high progesterone levels after day 100.

As may be expected from the discussion above, milk progesterone concentrations remain basal for a variable time after parturition (see Fig. 7.1a and b). Our milk progesterone studies have shown that the first ovulation is not usually accompanied by observable oestrus, and about 50% of first cycles tend to last for only about ten days (see Fig. 7.1a).

There has been much speculation as to the source and significance of this transient rise in progesterone concentrations. It has been suggested that such progesterone is secreted by a non-ovulated ovarian follicle that has undergone a degree of luteinization, or by a normal corpus luteum that is unable to respond maximally to the luteotrophic stimulus of luteinizing hormone (LH). It has also been suggested that this rise is preceded by an ovulation and that a premature release of $PGF_{2\alpha}$ from the uterus results in premature luteolysis (Manns *et al.*, 1983). In some postpartum situations, insulin levels may be sufficient to promote estradiol production, whilst IGF-I levels may not be sufficient to induce follicle proliferation. This may result in the ovulation of a small follicle, which in turn may produce a small corpus luteum (Wathes *et al.*, 2003), which could thus be of short duration.

The possibility exists that this first short cycle primes the endocrine system to secrete gonadotrophins so that normal ovarian cyclic function is then stimulated. However, the short cycle is not an essential prerequisite for normal cyclicity as all cows do not undergo it.

Although it is not normal for oestrus to be exhibited at the beginning of the first cycle, studies at the University of Nottingham have shown that both dairy and beef cows are able to conceive to service before any rise in milk progesterone concentrations (for example, see Fig. 7.1c). This phenomenon has been observed in a relatively high proportion of indigenous Shona and indigenous/exotic crossbred cows in Zimbabwe (P.J.H. Ball, personal observation). It thus appears that oestrous behaviour and ovulation can often precede any postpartum rise in progesterone concentrations (Manns *et al.*, 1983).

Factors affecting the postpartum acyclic period

Suckling

Many studies have shown that the onset of ovulation and/or oestrous behaviour can be delayed longer in both dairy and beef-type cows that suckle calves than in milked animals. Bulman & Lamming (1978) reported that dairy cows resumed ovarian cycles (as determined by milk progesterone measurements) after 24.0 ± 0.6 days postpartum. In our study of 2364 cows, over 80% had resumed ovarian cycles by day 30 postpartum and 95% by day 60. In suckling beef cows, however, the time to resumption of ovarian cycles was 59.9 ± 2.5 days after calving (Peters & Riley, 1982a) and there was considerably more variation both within and between herds.

Calf removal, either temporary or permanent, or the prevention of suckling by the fitting of nose-plates to the calves have been reported to shorten the acyclic period. Mastectomy of cows (removal of the udder) also shortens the acyclic period relative to non-suckling (Short *et al.*, 1972). This suggests that the presence of the udder itself may be inhibitory to ovarian activity, in addition to any specific effect of suckling.

Increasing the suckling intensity by double or multiple suckling (two or more calves per cow) has been reported to increase the postpartum acyclic period in some circumstances, although in our experiments we observed no difference between single- and double-suckled beef cows (Peters & Riley, 1982a). These experiments and those using the multiple-suckled Friesian cow as a model for the study of endocrine patterns in the postpartum anoestrous cow (Lamming *et al.*, 1981) have shown a wide variation in the length of the acyclic period from less than 15 days to in excess of 100 days. Varying the suckling intensity by restricting suckling to twice daily versus suckling ad libitum does not appear to affect the acyclic period significantly.

We showed that the pulsatile LH pattern reappears in milked dairy cows from about day 10 postpartum, whilst in the multiple-suckled Friesian cow it may not occur until day 50 or later (see Fig. 7.2). The situation in the single- or double-suckled beef cow appears to be intermediate between the two extremes. This is in line with suggestions that the onset of ovarian cycles is delayed in some suckling cows due to an inhibition of pulsatile LH release.

High prolactin concentrations inhibit ovarian activity in the human and in the ewe. They have also been implicated in the inhibition of ovarian activity in suckling cows, since it has been a widely held belief that suckling of calves induces hyperprolactinaemia. However, experiments have shown that plasma prolactin concentrations in suckling cows are no higher than those in milked or non-suckling cows. Furthermore, the pattern of gonadotrophin secretion in cows was not affected either by suppression of plasma prolactin concentrations with the dopamine agonist bromocryptine or by infusion of exogenous prolactin.

Milk yield

Associations between high milk yield and reduced fertility have been reported for many years, but whether reproductive performance is directly affected by milk yield remains debatable (Nebel & McGilliard, 1993). We have seen in Chapter 1 that increasing yields in the UK and USA have been reflected in reduced fertility, and longer acyclic periods have been observed in cows selected for high milk yield relative to control animals, but it is difficult to separate the effects of milk yield from other confounding factors, particularly that of nutritional status. For example, high-yielding cows in early lactation are often unable to maintain a state of positive energy balance despite high levels of feeding. In fact, Loeffler *et al.* (1999) and Grohn & Rajala-Schultz (2000) have stated that yield is not a risk factor for reproduction.

There is even less clear evidence as to the effect of milk yield on the time to onset of postpartum cyclicity. Again, milk yield is confounded with other factors, such as lactation number. First lactation cows produce less milk, but they eat less and have higher requirements for growth, so that their energy balance is different. When 400 dairy cows (half of which were in their first lactation, and assessed separately) were monitored using milk progesterone profiles there was a significant positive relationship between the interval to first ovulation and both peak and total milk yield.

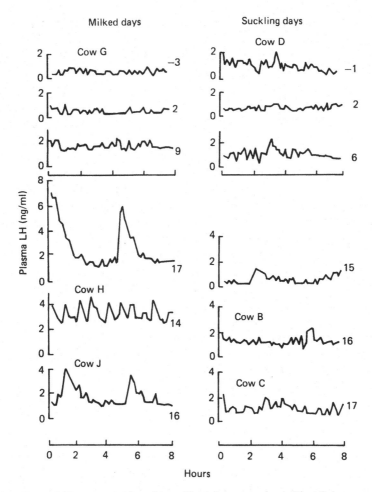

Fig. 7.2 Plasma LH concentrations in a milked dairy cow (cow G) at 3 days pre-partum and 2, 9 and 17 days postpartum and cows H and J on days 14 and 16 postpartum. Note presence of pulsatile patterns in the latter three profiles. Also shown are LH profiles for Friesian cows each suckling four calves; cow D on day 1 pre-partum, days 2, 6 and 15 postpartum, and cows B and C on days 16 and 17 postpartum, respectively. Note the absence of discrete pulsatile patterns.

Nutrition, body weight and body condition

The interaction between nutrition and overall fertility performance is very complex, and many experiments have produced conflicting results. Reviews include those of McClure (1994). The above discussion indicates the importance of nutrition in the initiation and maintenance of reproductive cycles and some of the mediating factors. The influence of nutrition is confounded with not only milk yield, but also many other factors, such as season and suckling. Energy intake appears to be more critical than protein intake in the mainte-nance of reproductive function as positive relationships between energy intake and reproductive performances have been demonstrated in several studies. Low energy intake in pre- and postpartum cows increases the length of the anoestrous period and in heifers has been shown to result in fewer ovarian follicles, lower progesterone levels and lower conception rates.

The use of body condition scoring techniques has played an important role in the monitoring of nutritional status in cattle (see Chapter 14). This technique, although somewhat subjective, is simple to perform, requires no specialized equipment and has the advantage that unlike body weight it is independent of skeletal size. Target body condition scores for cows at different stages of the reproductive/lactational cycle have been published and validated over many years (ADAS, 1978; Kilkenny, 1979; DEFRA, 2001) and are discussed in Chapter 14. Apart from effects on the acyclic period, nutritional status also appears to be critical in determining conception rate at mating. Positive relationships between nutritional status, body weight and body condition score and fertility in both dairy and beef cows have been documented (see Chapter 14). Although dietary energy supply is the most likely nutritional cause of poor reproductive performance, deficiency of other specific nutrients, particularly the vitamins and minerals, has been shown to affect fertility (see McClure, 1994).

Although the mechanisms involved are being elucidated, there is still much conflicting information on the relationship between nutrition and reproduction. It is, however, likely that energy balance is a prime factor determining the length of the acyclic period in dairy cows, and even in suckled beef cows long postpartum acyclic periods can be reduced by the provision of increased dietary energy. The individual interactions of nutritional status with ovarian activity, oestrous behaviour and fertility at mating still require more detailed study.

Season

In the temperate latitudes seasonal variations in conception rates and a longer interval between parturition and first oestrus in the winter and early spring have long been reported (e.g. Thibault *et al.*, 1966). Furthermore, spring-calving beef and dairy cows have been reported to undergo longer periods between calving and first ovulation than autumn calvers (Bulman & Lamming, 1978; Peters & Riley, 1982a).

Many wild species of Bovidae are seasonal breeders (Asdell, 1964), changes in daily photoperiod being the cue for onset or termination of ovarian activity. Thibault *et al.* (1966) suggested that photoperiod might play some role in seasonality of reproductive activity in the cow, and Peters & Riley (1982b) demonstrated a negative correlation between daily photoperiod during late pregnancy and the onset of ovarian cycles postpartum. It is thought that a vestigial sensitivity to photoperiod may be present in the domestic cow and that in feral cattle this pattern would predispose towards calving during the late spring to early summer, the optimal time for food supply. Season of birth has also been shown to affect age at first oestrus in heifers (see Chapter 4), with those born in spring reaching puberty approximately two months before those born in autumn.

Table 7.1 Relationship between body condition score and incidence of inactive ovaries in Holstein/Friesian and crossbred cows in Zimbabwe.

Location	No. of cows	Mean score	Percentage acyclic
Henderson[a]	65	2.03	21.3
Watsomba[b]	34	1.99	67.6

[a] Holstein–Friesian cows at Henderson Research Station.
[b] Crossbred cows on small-scale farms in the Watsomba area.

In hotter climates, seasonal anoestrus, short oestrous periods, poor conception rates and increased embryo mortality occur in both *Bos taurus* and *Bos indicus* during the hot season. Summer infertility due to heat stress is a well recognized phenomenon in such areas (Al-Katanani *et al.*, 1999), although embryo mortality may be the main specific problem (see Chapter 12). However, Sharpe & King (1981) suggested that prolonged anoestrus, often encountered when *Bos taurus* cattle are introduced into tropical environments, occurs mainly as a result of malnutrition rather than as a direct result of high temperatures.

In a study carried out by the Department of Research and Specialist services in Zimbabwe the incidence of ovarian acyclicity was measured using milk progesterone profiles in dairy cows including the Holstein/Friesian herd at Henderson Research Station as well as crossbred cows in the small-scale dairy sector. Many of the latter had extremely long periods of ovarian acyclicity, sometimes extending over several months (see Fig. 7.1c). A much lower proportion of the research herd cows were acyclic, even though their mean body condition score was only very slightly higher, as shown in Table 7.1.

This suggests that factors other than nutritional status were affecting the indigenous and crossbred cattle. Furthermore, most of these animals failed to start cycling at the onset of the rainy season. It was thought that suckling may have been one of the main reasons for delayed ovarian activity and this factor is being studied in more detail. These cattle may also be more sensitive to photoperiod than their more domesticated counterparts. This factor, superimposed on nutritional- and suckling-mediated delays to cycling, seems to favour calving after the onset of the following rainy season, usually after a two-year calving interval.

Uterine effects

Involution of the uterus is necessary before the cow can conceive again. The uteri of primiparous cows usually involute more rapidly than those of multiparous ones and suckling appears to stimulate involution, this usually being completed by about day 30 in the suckling cow. Eley *et al.* (1981) demonstrated a correlation between the duration of elevated plasma concentrations of the $PGF_{2\alpha}$ metabolite 13,14-dihydro-15 keto $PGF_{2\alpha}$ (PGFM) and time for completion of uterine involution. Furthermore, it has been shown that PGFM levels invariably return to baseline before any rise in progesterone occurs, suggesting that uterine involution is usually more or less complete before the first postpartum ovulation occurs. Dystocia may result in both long anoestrous periods postpartum and a decreased conception rate. Retained placenta may also result in longer postpartum acyclic periods. It is possible that these conditions may result in an inhibition of uterine involution thereby delaying ovulation. Other evidence suggests that lack of uterine involution predisposes to prolonged luteal function following the first postpartum ovulation (see Chapter 12).

The uterus has more specific effects on postpartum ovarian activity. Dominant follicles are less likely to be selected on the ovary ipsilateral to the previously pregnant uterine horn, but, if they are, the time to subsequent conception is reduced (Sheldon *et al.*, 2000). Bacterial contamination of the uterus after parturition is almost inevitable (Elliot *et al.*, 1968) and it is now thought that a high level of bacterial contamination can depress follicle selection, the effect usually being greatest in the previously pregnant horn (Sheldon *et al.*, 2002).

In summary, a variety of factors affect the onset of ovarian cycles in the postpartum period. Nutritional status, especially energy balance, seems to be the overriding factor, but suckling, milk yield and season can also be important. In many studies and in the practical situation, the effects of two or more of these factors may have been confounded. This has made it difficult to determine their relative importance in predicting the acyclic period. In many cases, especially in Third World conditions, the situation is further complicated by the fact that different breeds, within *Bos taurus*, *Bos indicus* and their crosses, vary in their tendency to postpartum acyclicity and in their response to specific factors affecting this. In practical terms it is apparent that, provided oestrus detection rates are satisfactory, then the acyclic period is unlikely to result in calving intervals greater than 365 days unless it is itself in excess of 50–60 days.

Induction of ovulation in postpartum cows

We have shown how the inhibitory effects of the environmental factors discussed above on the reproductive system are mediated by the endocrine system and probably via a common final mechanism. The availability of hormonal therapy that would overcome acyclicity or true anoestrus, irrespective of primary cause, would be of great advantage, particularly in beef cattle where husbandry and nutrition are often only marginally adequate. In the past many such treatments have been based on empirical approaches with little regard to the underlying reproductive physiology. However, detailed knowledge of the pattern of hormone release is essential in order to understand the mechanisms controlling ovulation and ovarian cycles so that appropriate treatments can be designed. It is only since the relatively recent development of radioimmunoassay (RIA) techniques for hormone measurement that detailed patterns of hormone release have been described in cows.

Gonadotrophins

Several workers have attempted to induce ovulation and ovarian cycles in cows using the exogenous gonadotrophins, pregnant mare's serum gonadotrophin (PMSG) and human chorionic gonadotrophin (HCG), since early work in the 1940s showed that the bovine ovary is sensitive to these compounds. Results have been very variable since some animals do not respond, some ovulate and then revert to anoestrus and PMSG induces multiple ovulations in a proportion of cases depending on the dose used.

Gonadotrophin releasing hormone (GnRH)

GnRH injection of cattle induces release of both LH and FSH. Moreover, as mentioned above, the responsiveness of the anterior pituitary to GnRH stimulation increases during the early postpartum period, being maximal by about day 12 in dairy cows and by days 20–30 in suckling cows. There have been many attempts to induce ovulation in postpartum cows by single intramuscular injections of 100–500 mg GnRH and these have given variable results. In a study at the University of Nottingham, the calving to conception interval was not significantly reduced in GnRH-injected cows as compared to controls (see Chapter 12, Table 12.3). In order to apply these treatments in practice, more consistent responses would be necessary.

At the above dose levels of GnRH, LH release of pre-ovulatory surge magnitude usually occurs, depending on the responsiveness of the pituitary. However, ovarian follicles appear to require a two- to three-day period of rising plasma LH concentrations in order to mature fully prior to ovulation (see Chapter 4). A pre-ovulatory LH surge will therefore induce ovulation only if a follicle at the appropriate stage of development is already present. Alternatively, the induced LH release might result in premature luteinization of an unovulated follicle and transient secretion of progesterone sufficient to initiate ovarian cycles.

As a gradual increase in LH concentrations and pulse frequency occurs prior to ovulation during the natural cycle (see Chapter 4) and before the first ovulation postpartum, a more logical approach to the induction of ovulation might be to induce this pattern of LH secretion using very small doses of GnRH, or alternatively to stimulate it using exogenous LH.

There have been numerous attempts to induce ovulation consistently using controlled release formulations of GnRH, but our approach has been to attempt to induce LH release as in the early follicular phase of the ovarian cycle and that seen in postpartum cows prior to the first ovulation. Repeated injections of 5 mg GnRH were given intravenously at two-hourly intervals for 48 hours to postpartum beef cows. A pulsatile pattern of LH secretion occurred in response to treatment and four out of five cows ovulated and underwent ovarian cycles (Riley *et al.*, 1981). The question remains as to whether the pulsatile mode of GnRH administration is important per se or whether a constant administration of the same total dose would achieve the same result. If this were so then it might be possible to develop either a slow release depot injection or implant containing GnRH. Experiments are continuing to investigate these possibilities and are currently showing promise, but there has been little success in terms of development of a reliable commercial project.

Progesterone

Progesterone suppresses the release of LH and its withdrawal results in a gradual rise in plasma LH concentrations, culminating in a pre-ovulatory LH surge occurring in cows that respond, approximately 48 hours afterwards. The action of exogenous progesterone whether natural or synthetic may be considered as a simulation of the natural luteal phase or at least the first short progesterone cycle described earlier in this chapter.

Early work on the use of progesterone to induce ovulation postpartum produced equivocal results. Some authors reported a delay in the onset of ovarian cycles whilst others reported that progesterone (with or without oestrogen) advanced the time of the first ovulation. Invariably, however, fertility at the induced oestrus was low. It has been shown in the sheep at least that long periods of progesterone administration adversely affect sperm transport in the female genital tract.

Roche *et al.* (1981) reported that treatment of beef cows with the progesterone-releasing intravaginal device for 12 days resulted in ovulation in about half of the cows treated. Peters (1982) reported that the calving to conception interval of progesterone-releasing intravaginal device (PRID)-treated beef cows was reduced only if used before day 30 postpartum. Mulvehill & Sreenan (1977) reported the best success in induction of ovulation in beef cows by injecting 750 international units of PMSG at the time of progesterone withdrawal. In the dairy cow, Ball & Lamming (1983) and Drew *et al.* (1982) have reported a reduction in the calving to conception interval of up to 14 days following the use of PRID (see Table 12.3). None of these treatments has been widely applied commercially, mainly because of the variable success rates reported.

Conclusion

To conclude this chapter, it should be said that an understanding of the endocrinology of the postpartum period is essential for the development of hormone therapy to overcome delays in the onset of ovarian activity. No completely successful treatment has yet been devised, but this continues to be an active area of research. If the underlying cause of delay is the stress and negative energy balance of early lactation, then it is possible that no hormonal treatment can be completely successful, or even desirable.

References

Adam, C.L., Gadd, T.S., Findlay, P.A. & Wathes, D.C. (2000) *Journal of Endocrinology*, **166**, 247–254.

ADAS (1978) *Advisory Leaflet 612*.

Al-Katanani, Y.M., Webb, D.W. & Hansen, P.J. (1999) *Journal of Dairy Science*, **82**, 2611–2616.

Armstrong, D.G., Gong, J.G. & Webb, R. (2003) *Reproduction Supplement*, **61**, 403–414.

Asdell, S.A. (1964) *Patterns of Mammalian Reproduction*, 2nd edn. Constable, London.

Ball, P.J.H. & Lamming, G.E. (1983) *British Veterinary Journal*, **139**, 522–527.

Beam, S.W. & Butler, W.R. (1999) *Journal of Reproduction and Fertility* (Suppl. 54), 411–424.

Bulman, D.C. (1979) *British Veterinary Journal*, **135**, 460.

Bulman, D.C. & Lamming, G.E. (1978) *Journal of Reproduction and Fertility*, **54**, 447.

Butler, W.R. (2001) *British Society of Animal Science Occasional Publication*, **26**, 133–146.

DEFRA (2001) *Action on Animal Health and Welfare Leaflet. Condition Scoring of Dairy Cows.*

Diskin, M.G., Mackey, D.R., Roche, J.F. & Sreenan, J.M. (2003) *Animal Reproduction Science*, **78**, 345–370.

Drew, S.B, Gould, C.M., Dawson, P.L.L. & Altman, J.F.B. (1982) *Veterinary Record*, **111**, 103.

Eley, D.S., Thatcher, W.W., Head, N.H., Collier, R.J., Wilcox, C.I. & Call, E.P. (1981) *Journal of Dairy Science*, **64**, 312.

Elliot, L., McMahon, K.J., Gier, H.Y. & Marion, G.B. (1968) *American Journal of Veterinary Research*, **29**, 77–81.

Grohn, Y.H. & Rajala-Schultz, P.J. (2000) *Animal Reproduction Science*, **60–61**, 605–614.

Kadokawa, H., Blache, D., Yamada, Y. & Martin, G.B. (2000) *Reproduction, Fertility and Development*, **12**, 405–411.

Kilkenny, J.B. (1979) *World Review of Animal Production*, **14**, 65.

Lamming, G.E., Wathes, D.C. & Peters, A.R. (1981) *Journal of Reproduction and Fertility* (Suppl. 30), 155.

Lamming, G.E., Darwash, A.O., Wathes, D.C. & Ball, P.J.H. (1998) *Journal of the Royal Agricultural Society of England*, **159**, 82–93.

Loeffler, S.H., de Vries, M.J. & Schukken, Y.H. (1999) *Journal of Dairy Science*, **82**, 2589–2604.

Manns, J.G., Humphrey, W.D., Flood, P.F., Mapletoft, R.J., Rawlings, N. & Cheng, K.W. (1983) *Canadian Journal of Animal Science*, **63**, 331.

McClure, T.J. (1994) *Nutritional and Metabolic Infertility in the Cow*. CAB International, Wallingford.

Mulvehill, P. & Sreenan, J.M. (1977) *Journal of Reproduction and Fertility*, **50**, 323.

Nebel, R.L. & McGilliard, M.L. (1993) *Journal of Dairy Science*, **76**, 3257–3268.

Peters, A.R. (1982) *Veterinary Record,* **110,** 515.

Peters, A.R. & Riley, G.M. (1982a) *Animal Production,* **34,** 145.

Peters, A.R. & Riley, G.M. (1982b) *British Veterinary Journal,* **138,** 533.

Riley, G.M., Peters, A.R. & Lamming, G.E. (1981) *Journal of Reproduction and Fertility,* **63,** 559.

Roche, J.F. & Diskin, M.G. (2001) *British Society of Animal Science Occasional Publication,* **26,** 31–42.

Roche, J.F., Ireland, J.J. & Mawhinney, S. (1981) *Journal of Reproduction and Fertility* (Suppl. 30), 211.

Sharpe, P.H. & King, G.I. (1981) *Journal of Dairy Science,* **64,** 672.

Sheldon, I.M., Noakes, D.E. & Dobson, H. (2000) *Theriogenology,* **54,** 409–419.

Sheldon, I.M., Noakes, D.E., Rycroft, A.N., Pfeiffer, D.U. & Dobson, H. (2002) *Reproduction,* **123,** 837–845.

Short, R.E., Bellows, R.A., Moody, E.L. & Howland, B.E. (1972) *Journal of Animal Science,* **34,** 70.

Snyder, J.L., Clapper, J.A., Roberts, A.J., Sanson, D.W., Hamernik, D.L. & Moss, G.E. (1999) *Biology of Reproduction,* **61,** 219–224.

Spicer, L.J. & Echternkamp, S.E. (1995) *Domestic Animal Endocrinology,* **12,** 223–245.

Thibault, C., Courot, M., Martinet, L., Mauleon, P., De Mesnil du Buisson, F., Ortovant, R., Pelletier, J. & Signoret, J.P. (1966) *Journal of Animal Science* (Suppl. 25), 119.

Wathes, D.C., Taylor, V.J., Cheng, Z. & Mann, G.E. (2003) *Reproduction* (Suppl. 61), 1–19.

Webb, R., Lamming, G.E., Haynes, N.B., Hafs, H.D. & Manns, J.O. (1977) *Journal of Reproduction and Fertility,* **50,** 203.

Chapter 8
Oestrous Behaviour and Its Detection

Introduction

The oestrous period in a cow is that time during which she will stand to be mounted by a bull or another cow. Changes in the levels of circulating hormones, particularly oestradiol from the developing follicle, induce the behavioural changes associated with oestrus (see Chapter 4). These changes may begin one or two days before standing oestrus. The cow will become more likely to mount other cows that are in oestrus, and other cows in the herd will begin to take an interest in her – sniffing her and resting their chins on her back, for example. Standing oestrus normally persists for several hours (see Table 4.2). There also seems to be a tendency for a higher proportion of oestrous activity to occur at night. The main period of oestrous activity precedes ovulation by approximately 12–15 hours. Although natural service normally occurs during standing oestrus, artificial insemination is most successful during the last half of and up to around six hours after standing oestrus (Asdell, 1964). The events around the time of oestrus are summarized in Fig. 8.1.

Artificial insemination is probably used in only 3–5% of beef cows in the UK (data calculated from MMB, 1982 and MLC, 1983). The main reason for this lack of usage is the practical difficulty of detecting oestrus in extensively managed suckler herds. Consequently most beef breeders use a bull both to detect oestrus and to breed with the cows. Most of the information in this chapter therefore relates to dairy herds.

Unless a bull is to be left running with the herd it is essential that stockpersons know when oestrus is occurring so that the cow can be taken to the bull, or artificial insemination carried out, at the optimum time for fertilization to occur. This means that efficient and accurate detection of oestrus, or at least of changes associated with ovulation, is of vital importance.

As was discussed in Chapter 1, a cow's calving interval is influenced mainly by the calving to conception interval, which is influenced in turn by a number of factors including the occurrence and detection of oestrus at the correct time. Milk progesterone profile studies have consistently shown that the majority of the cows experience normal ovarian cycles by the time that insemination is desired, but that only about 50% of ovulations are accompanied by a reported observed oestrus. In a study at Nottingham University, oestrus was observed by herdspeople in only 60% of approximately 2500 cows in commercial herds

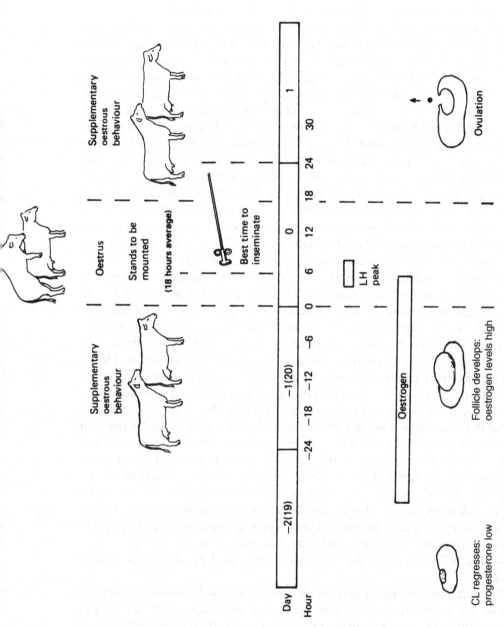

Fig. 8.1 Events around the time of oestrus in the cow.

by the time they had reached 60 days postpartum. Fifteen per cent of the cows were not observed in oestrus during the critical period after 50 days postpartum even though they were cycling normally. This indicates that oestrus detection problems are a major cause of extended calving intervals.

The worsening problem is due in part to increasing pressures on stockpersons who are able to spend less time on detecting and recording oestrus. However, there also seems to have been a decline in the intensity of oestrous behaviour in recent years. In Chapter 12, we will discuss the nutritional and other stress factors that affect the reproductive system and contribute to problems of ovarian cyclicity, fertilization and conceptus survival. A specific effect of energy deficiency and stress is a suppression of oestradiol production by the dominant follicle. This could in turn affect the intensity of oestrous behaviour and help to explain the apparent drop in oestrus intensity in modern dairy herds. Lyimo *et al.* (2000) found a high correlation between blood oestradiol levels and the intensity of oestrous behaviour. Records from more than 244 000 cows in more than 2100 herds were collected as part of the ADAS 'Datamate' computer-based reproductive management program for about ten years from 1986. They showed that 57% of Friesian cows were inseminated within 20 days of their start of service date, compared to 50% of Holsteins.

If a given opportunity to inseminate a cow is missed because of a failure to detect oestrus, that cow's calving interval will be extended by at least another cycle length (i.e., about 21 days), unless ovulation is artificially induced (see Chapter 7). The financial losses associated with these extended calving intervals have also been discussed in Chapter 1. It is thus easy to see that the economic consequences of missing oestrus can be extremely important. On the other hand, there can be serious consequences if oestrus is recorded at a time other than around ovulation. At best the falsely recorded oestrus could mislead the herdsperson as to when the next true oestrus is due. If the cow is inseminated the cost will be wasted. Furthermore, when the uterus is under the influence of progesterone as it is during the luteal phase of pregnancy, it has a very low resistance to pathogens, so that infection could result from the mistimed insemination. At worst, if the cow is already pregnant, insemination into the uterus could cause her to abort. Such abortions have been detected in studies using milk progesterone profiles. Studies at the Scottish Agricultural College (SAC) have revealed a number of such cases, in spite of previous publicity about the dangers of inseminating cows that could possibly already be pregnant. Fig. 8.2 summarizes the incidence of mistimed inseminations in these studies.

The trend towards larger dairy herds and an increased reliance on employed labour has added to the problems of oestrus detection to the extent that many farmers are reverting to the use of a bull for natural service with at least some of their cows. An understanding of the characteristics of oestrus, procedures for its detection and a knowledge of possible aids to oestrus detection are therefore of paramount importance in achieving efficient reproductive performance.

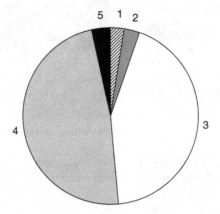

1	Abnormal (acyclic, cystic, etc.)	2.7% of inseminations
2	Mid cycle	2.5%
3	Correct timing, but failed to conceive	43%
4	Correct timing – pregnant	48.5%
5	Cow already pregnant	3.3%

Fig. 8.2   Timing of AI (percentage of AI carried out at various times) as subsequently revealed by milk progesterone profiles.

Characteristics of oestrus

The main criterion

For the stockperson, the only reliable indication of oestrus is that the cow will stand to be mounted by a bull or another cow (Fig. 8.3a) and can often be seen 'soliciting' or apparently encouraging other cows to mount her (Fig. 8.3b). A cow in oestrus is often described as being 'in heat' or 'bulling'.

From the point of view of oestrus detection, it is fortunate that other cows, especially if they are also within a few days of oestrus, will mount a cow in oestrus. In the wild this characteristic possibly served to draw the bull's attention to the oestrous cow, and likewise this may also draw the stockperson's attention to the appropriate cow. In fact, the most frequently observed sign of oestrus is that the cow tries to mount other cows. This probably accounts for the common mistake of thinking that the cow being mounted is the one in oestrus. If an oestrous cow tries to mount a non-oestrous cow she is usually unsuccessful unless the other cow is trapped, or is mounted from the front or the side so that she cannot escape. In Fig. 8.3c, for example, it is possible that the mounting cow is the one in oestrus since the other cow is trying to walk away. Oestrous cows sometimes manage to mount others that are trapped by fences or other cows, or that find it difficult to escape because of illness, injury or even fear of cows higher in the pecking order. This can be

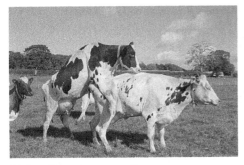

(a) Standing to be mounted[1]

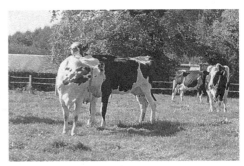

(b) 'Soliciting' another cow to mount

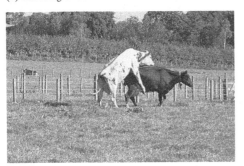

(c) Mounted, but trying to escape[2]

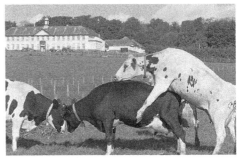

(d) Aggression[3]

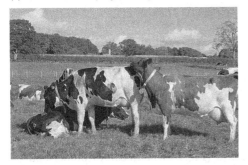

(e) Chin resting

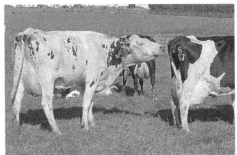

(f) Vulval sniffing

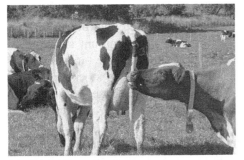

(g) Flehman lip curl

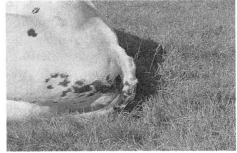

(h) Ruffled hair[4]

[1] This was the first mount after 45 minutes' observation!

[2] The mounted cow was not in standing heat, but was due shortly.

[3] The same black cow, too busy fighting to avoid being mounted.

[4] A sign that the cow has been mounted.

Fig. 8.3 Behavioural signs of oestrus in the cow.

misleading. Normally, the oestrous cow will only be mounted from the rear by other cows, but she will attempt to mount her herd mates from the front, the rear or the side.

Supplementary signs of oestrus

There are a number of supplementary behavioural signs of oestrus which in themselves may not mean that a cow is due for insemination, but they could be useful in drawing attention to particular animals. The main signs are summarized below:

Signs that the cow has been mounted
- Dirty rump and flanks.
- Ruffled hair on the tail-head (Fig. 8.3h). Sometimes patches of hair are completely removed and the skin may be raw or bleeding.
- Streaks of saliva or signs of licking on her flanks from interested herd mates.

Other behavioural changes
- Aggressiveness (Fig. 8.3d).
- Bellowing.
- Restlessness.
- 'Flehmen lip curl'. This may be displayed by the cow in oestrus or, more frequently, a cow that is interested in her (Fig. 8.3g).
- Other departures from routine, such as a cow coming into the milking parlour last when she would normally be one of the first, or vice versa. At pasture, she and one or more others particularly interested in her could be the only ones not grazing.

Physiological changes
- Increased mucus secretion in the cervix and vagina. This leads to another common and quite reliable sign of oestrus: the clear string of mucus that is extruded from the vagina and often adheres to the tail. The cow is often said to have a 'bulling string' or to be 'sliming'. In some cases, such as when cows are continually tied up, this may be the main or only criterion for having them inseminated. However, the timing of expulsion of mucus is variable and insemination could be mistimed by up to two days. If the mucus is cloudy or discoloured, the vagina could well be infected and the cow is not necessarily in oestrus.
- At times, especially in cold weather, vapour can be seen rising from the backs of cows in oestrus. This results from a rise in body temperature associated either with increased activity or with the physiological changes of oestrus.
- In dairy cows there is commonly a drop in milk yield on the day of oestrus, which may be due either to reduced production or to an interference with the let-down process. The basic cause could be psychological stress or

physiological change. As there are many other causes of reduced milk yield, it is not in itself a very good indication of oestrus.

- If the lips of the vulva are parted they are usually more swollen and a deeper red in colour in an oestrous as compared with a non-oestrous cow.

- Around two days after the end of oestrus, blood or bloody mucus is often seen extruding from the vagina or adhering to the skin around the vulva or on the tail. This results from the increased secretion of blood products (including the white cells that help to combat infection) into the uterine lumen under the influence of oestradiol at oestrus. Stockpeople sometimes assume that a cow is not pregnant if she 'bleeds', but in fact the occurrence of this metoestrous bleeding is independent of insemination and conception.

Guidelines for oestrus detection

Obviously, oestrus detection will not be effective if the cow does not display clear signs that she is in oestrus. A poorly fed, sick, cold, wet or bullied cow is much less likely to show heat signs. The environment should also be conducive to activity and to ease of observation. Generally speaking, oestrus is better displayed when the cows are out of doors. When cows are housed, floors should not be slippery, and there should be enough room to move around and interact with interested herd mates. If a self-feed silage clamp is in use, the area in front of it is useful in this regard; if not, a loafing area should be provided. The building should be well lit, and planned to give good views of the cows.

Standing oestrus may persist for as little as two hours, with a tendency for a higher proportion of oestrous activity to occur at night. There is thus a greater probability of detecting oestrus if observations are carried out frequently, and if a late evening check is made. It is usually recommended that four or five checks be made each day. This also makes it easier to determine the time of onset of true standing oestrus and thus have a better idea when to inseminate. Supplementary signs such as mucus secretion and attempting to mount other cows are more variable in their time of onset and duration and are normally of little use in determining insemination times.

It is difficult to give a hard and fast rule on the length of time required to watch the cows. The more often and the longer cows are observed, the more heats are likely to be detected. The cow in Fig. 8.3a, for example, was watched for nearly 45 minutes before she was mounted, and intervals between mounts are often up to 20 minutes long. Any extra help with detection is therefore always welcome, but inexperienced helpers should be properly instructed and supervised to make sure they know what they are looking for. If in doubt, advice on oestrus detection can be obtained from advisory or extension services or from veterinary surgeons.

When checking for oestrus it is sometimes helpful to get the cows moving and thus initiate activity, but it is normally best to observe them quietly for a while without distracting them. Thus, for example, a stockperson should not send his/her dog to round up the cows until they have been observed for oestrus, and during winter lights should be left on all evening so that cows are not disturbed by lights being switched on during a late evening check.

To summarize:

• Observe for oestrus frequently and for sufficient time. A cow in heat may only be mounted every 15 or 20 minutes. Five minutes will not do!
• Late evening (from about 8–10 pm) checks are very important.
• The cows and their environment should be in the right condition.
• Good records are vital to keep track of regular oestrus cycles and to highlight irregular ones.

Records from 'Datamate' confirm the importance of good oestrus detection procedures, as the results in Table 8.1 show.

Oestrus detection score

Van Eerdenburg *et al.* (1996) recorded the various signs of oestrus and composed a scale according to the frequency of these symptoms during and between oestrous periods. Each oestrous symptom was given a score and the scores were summed for a 24-hour period. If a score of >100 points was reached within a 24-hour period, the cow was considered to be in oestrus. Standing was

Table 8.1 Factors affecting submission rate [percentage served within 20 days of start of service date (SSD)].

	No. of herds	No. of cows	Served within 20 days of SSD	
			(No.)	*(%)*
Frequency of observation				
No set routine	438	48694	24595	51
Once or twice daily	405	40013	19472	49
Three times a day	617	70086	37727	54
Four or more times a day	672	86185	52648	61
Latest observation				
Before 8 pm	194	17655	8134	46
8–10 pm	1094	122938	67290	55
After 10 pm	844	104205	59018	57
Housing				
Winter housed	2104	241647	132892	55
Year-round housed	26	3016	1468	49
Outwintered	2	135	82	61

observed to accompany only 37% of ovulations (as detected by daily milk progesterone measurements), but the use of this scale and observing the herd twice daily for 30 minutes resulted in a detection rate of 74% with no incorrect assessments. Van Eerdenburg *et al.* (2002) reported a significant correlation (0.31) between detection score and the day of ovulation.

In a subsequent study at The University of Reading's Centre for Dairy Research (CEDAR), Pearse and Bleach (pers. comm.) used the scoring system described by Van Eerdenburg *et al.*, but with a threshold of 50 points within 24 hours. A group of 45 cows was observed three times daily for 30 minutes. Overall, 73% of all ovulations were preceded by oestrus (i.e., the cow had a point score of greater than 50 within 24 hours). However, of the 136 occasions when the behavioural score of a cow exceeded 50 points, 21 (15%) were not associated with ovulation (i.e., 'false positives' occurring in the luteal phase).

Aids to oestrus detection

Records

Without doubt, the most important aid to oestrus detection is an effective, even if simple, recording system. Firstly, it is important that stockpeople carry with them a diary or a small notebook to make a note of observations such as cows in heat, which may otherwise be forgotten by the time they return to the office or dairy. A simple code can be used to save time and space. If 257 mounts 621, for example, 257/621 could be written in the notebook or diary. A message board, such as the blackboard shown in Fig. 8.4, can be a useful way of ensuring that the person responsible for insemination is aware of sightings by other farm staff.

The basic requirement of fertility recording is to record every insemination and every occurrence of oestrus, even if the cow in question is not due to be served. This information should then be used to predict when the cow is next due in heat so that she can be watched extra-carefully around that time (but not ignored at other times!). Conversely, if it is suspected that a cow may be in heat, checking back to see if she was in heat approximately 21 days previously will help to establish the fact. Signs of metoestrous bleeding, indicating that the cow was in oestrus approximately two days previously, should also be recorded for future reference.

Records of oestrous activity will also help to draw attention to cows with frequent and/or irregular heats, which may need veterinary attention. A simple and effective aid in this respect is a 21-day calendar, such as is shown in Fig. 8.5.

As an adjunct to good record keeping it is important that all the cows are clearly identified so that there is never any doubt as to which one is actually in oestrus.

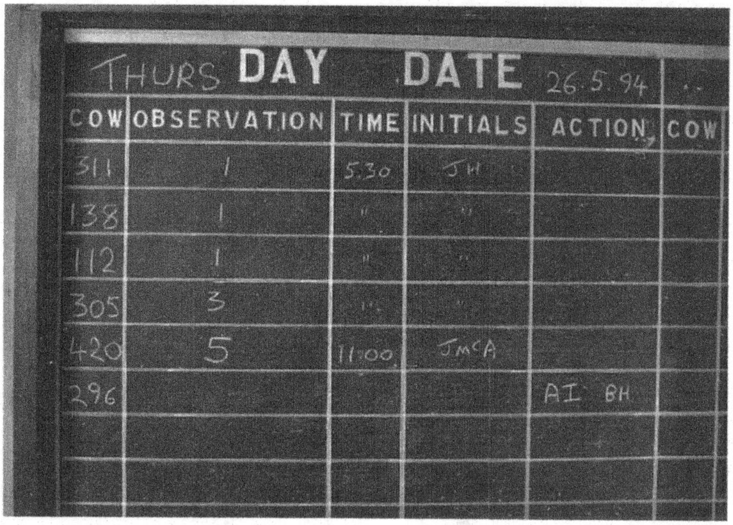

Fig. 8.4 Message board for recording oestrous observations. Codes indicate observation (e.g., 1 = standing to be mounted).

Heat mount detectors

These devices give the stockperson a visual indication that a cow has been ridden by one or more others. One such type is illustrated in Fig. 8.6. It consists of a cylindrical plastic container of red dye inside a clear plastic capsule. The cylinder is hidden by an opaque cover under the capsule, so that the red colour is only seen after the dye has been squeezed out of the cylinder by pressure from a mounting cow. The whole unit is mounted on a canvas patch, which is glued to the cow's back in the position shown. Once triggered, the device has to be replaced to aid detection of subsequent oestrous events.

Attempts have been made to devise reusable detectors. One such device incorporates a small plastic 'flag' which erects when the device is triggered and is designed to be pushed back into the prone position for retriggering at a subsequent oestrus. Reports from farmers suggest, however, that the device is not sufficiently robust to survive more than one oestrus!

Tail paste provides a cheaper alternative, which can be very effective under the right conditions. Original studies in New Zealand used commercially available emulsion paints, but these proved less satisfactory under British conditions and with some brands there may be a danger of a skin reaction or poisoning if the paint is licked. Formulations have thus been devised specifically for oestrus detection in cattle and marketed versions have included a thixotropic paste which is worked well into the hair on the tail-head to form a strip about 20 cm long and 5 cm wide along the midline. The paste dries rapidly to form a hard cake, which breaks up and is rubbed off after several mounts by other cows. Experiments in one experimental and several commercial herds (Ball *et al.*,

16	6	27	17	10	31	21	12	2
17	7	28	18	11	April 1	22	13	3
18	8	29	19	12	2	23	14	4
19	9	30	20	13	3	24	15	5
20	10	31	21	14	4	25	16	6
21	11	February 1	22	15	5	26	17	7
22	12	2 *15*	23	16	6	27	18	8
23	13	3	24	17	7	28	19	9
24	14	4 *101 AI*	25	18	8	29	20	10
25	15 *101*	5	26 *101 N.S.*	19	9	30	21	11
26	16	6	27 *6*	20	10	May 1	22	12
27	17	7	28	21	11	2	23	13
28	18	8	March 1	22	12	3	24	14
29	19	9	2	23	13	4	25	15
30	20	10 *24*	3	24	14	5	26	16
31	21	11	4	25	15	6	27	17
January 1	2	12	5	26	16	7	28	18
2 *6 CALVED*	23	13 *53 26*	6	27	17	8	29	19
3 *26*	24 *26 AI*	14	7	28	18	9	30	20
4	25	15	8	29	19	10	31	21
5 *24 CALVED*	26	16	9	30	20	11	June 1	22

Fig. 8.5 A 21-day calendar for recording oestrus. This shows at a glance that cow 24, for example, recorded in oestrus on 10 February, is due again on 3 March.

1983) showed that tail paste correctly identified significantly more oestrous periods than did stockpeople during their routine observations. More recently available alternatives include at least one spray can version. We are unaware of any scientific evaluation of its efficacy, but we felt, as did the farm staff, that it was less satisfactory than the paste.

There is a danger with both heat mount detectors and tail pastes or paints that they may be triggered accidentally on a non-oestrous cow. In contrast to the findings of Ball *et al.* (1983), Ducker *et al.* (1983) reported an unacceptably high incidence of tail paste being rubbed off at the wrong time. The efficacy of detectors or paste will vary with different herds under different housing and

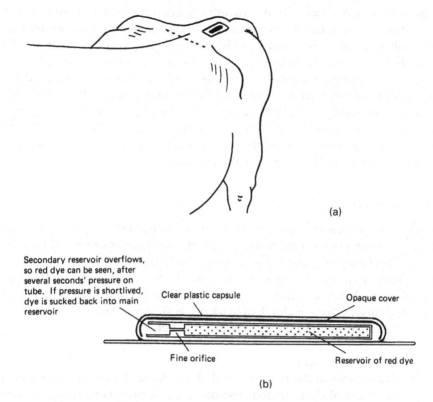

Secondary reservoir overflows, so red dye can be seen, after several seconds' pressure on tube. If pressure is shortlived, dye is sucked back into main reservoir

Clear plastic capsule

Opaque cover

Fine orifice

Reservoir of red dye

(a)

(b)

Fig. 8.6 Heat mount detector. (a) Position of detector or tail paste. (b) Details of heat mount detector.

management systems, but normally they should not be relied on as the sole means of determining when to inseminate. They are likely to be of most value for individual problem cows.

A number of electronic heat mount detectors have been developed. They count the number of times a cow is mounted. The use of one of these, a real-time radiotelometric system, which provides data on the time and duration of each mount, was reported by Stevenson *et al.* (1996). Rorie *et al.* (2002) compared such a system with less expensive stand-alone mount monitors, which also provide the necessary information for optimum timing of insemination, but are more labour intensive. The additional cost of such devices is unlikely to be justified in terms of improved performance (Mottram & Frost, 1997).

Closed-circuit television

Given suitably confined housing, or a loafing area where sexually active cows can be relied upon to congregate, television, film or video cameras can be effective in helping to spot cows in oestrus. A night's activities can be played back at high speed and the action slowed or 'frozen' to identify cows displaying oestrous activity. Alternatively, passive infra-red detectors can be used to switch on the camera. These can be set to scan above cow height, so that they are triggered only when there is mounting activity. The system obviously relies heavily on the stockperson knowing his/her cows well, or having them very clearly identified. Video systems designed to monitor cows due to calve and to aid the detection of cows in oestrus are now available commercially. The cost of such systems is continually being reduced, and can sometimes be justified when balanced against the returns from improved oestrus detection. Furthermore, they can be used to monitor cows in the process of calving and sick cows, and this convenience can also help to justify the expense.

Teaser animals

In this context, 'teasers' are any other animals that take an interest in an oestrous cow and in so doing help to make the stockperson aware of her. For the most part they are other cows, bulls or steers that are sexually aggressive so that they are inclined to mount, and thus identify, oestrous cows. They are more effective if they are equipped with some device for marking the mounted cows. One such device – a chin ball marker – is shown in Fig. 8.7.

Teaser animals fall into the categories listed below:

(1) Cows, bulls and steers
   • Other cows in the herd. Cows that are themselves in or near oestrus are more likely to mount oestrous cows. A nymphomaniac cow, with cystic follicles, is often very effective at picking out cows in oestrus. The condition is sometimes difficult to cure, and if all hope of return

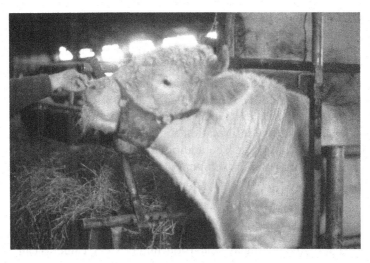

Fig. 8.7   Bull wearing a chin ball marker. (Courtesy of Department of Animal Science and Production, University College Dublin.)

to normal has been abandoned, it may be worth keeping the cow for some time and making use of her oestrus-detecting abilities before she is finally sold.

- Vasectomized bulls. In common with intact bulls these animals can be aggressive, so that there is a risk of injury to cows or personnel and there is the possibility of spread of venereal disease.
- Androgenized steers. These can also spread venereal disease and are likely to be even more aggressive than vasectomized bulls.
- Surgically modified bulls. Various treatments have been attempted to prevent intromission, so that teaser bulls would not spread venereal disease. These include penectomy, penis deviation and a device in the prepuce to prevent erection. These animals are likely to lose their libido after they have been used for some time and in any case most of these methods are unacceptable because of animal welfare considerations.

A common drawback of the various types of teasers listed is that they tend to cultivate favourites among oestrous cows and may completely ignore others that are also in oestrus. If there is already a bull on the farm it is helpful to house him near the cows. A cow in oestrus is liable to seek out the bull and thus identify herself.

(2) Other species. There have been occasional instances of interaction with other species, such as horses and goats, which have been used on farms to draw attention to oestrous cows. However, dogs are the only animals to which serious consideration has been given to their potential for oestrus detection in cattle. Experiments in the United States Department of Agriculture (Kiddy *et al.*, 1978) have shown that it is possible for dogs to detect oestrus if they have been trained to recognize the scent of vaginal swabs from oestrous cows. There are many practical difficulties, and the use of dogs is unlikely to be put to widespread use, but the idea has been further researched as a possible means of determining the chemical involved and thus devising a more objective means of detecting it in the oestrous cow.

Movement detectors

A cow in heat tends to be more restless than usual. The increased movement associated with oestrus has been measured experimentally by means of pedometers strapped to the cows' hind legs (Kiddy, 1977). Maatje *et al.* (1997) found that the chance of conception was highest between 6 and 17 hours after increased pedometer activity, the estimated optimum being 11.8 hours. Pedometers are now available commercially. Rorie *et al.* (2002) considered that of all the commercially available electronic oestrus detection devices, pedometers were the most applicable to lactating dairy cattle and that they had greater accuracy and efficiency when combined with visual observation.

It is more difficult to observe oestrous activity in cows that are tied up in cowsheds. Preliminary work at Nottingham University has suggested the possibility of measuring the increased restlessness of such cows when they are in oestrus by means of a counter activated by a doppler-type intruder detector.

Temperature measurement

It has been known for many decades that there are changes in body temperature associated with oestrus in the cow. Body temperature tends to drop one or two days before oestrus and to rise again to a short-lived peak on the day of oestrus. Preliminary experiments at Nottingham University have suggested that the peaks may be associated with the pre-ovulatory luteinizing hormone rise. Experiments in the Netherlands, USA and the UK (see Ball *et al.*, 1978) have shown that it is possible to detect oestrus-related temperature changes in milk, using sensors in milking machine clusters. These changes are very small compared to normal temperature fluctuations within and between cows, and initial investigations into their use in oestrus detection in practice have been disappointing (Fordham, 1984). The accurate measurements possible with modern electronics, combined with judicious analysis of the data, give rise to the possibility of using automatic temperature measurements as an oestrus detection aid, if only as an adjunct to other measurements. However, even such combined measures are unlikely to achieve sufficient oestrus detection accuracy (Mottram & Frost, 1997).

Body temperature changes have also been transmitted from sensors implanted in the ear or under the skin (Maatje & Rossing, personal communication), but the drawbacks in terms of cost and possible discomfort to the animals probably outweigh the advantages.

Vaginal resistance measurements

During oestrus there is an increase in the volume and ionic content of vaginal mucus, so that it is better able to conduct electricity. Various probes have been designed to measure the consequent fall in electrical resistance in the vagina (e.g., Heckman *et al.*, 1979). This fall normally lasts for no more than 24 hours, so that for routine oestrus detection the probe would have to be inserted daily into each cow's vagina. This would be impractical and liable to cause inflammation. Studies at Nottingham University showed that variation between cows can be as great as oestrus-related changes in individual cows. Technical development has continued, and a vaginal probe based on the principle is currently available in the UK. However, there is no getting around the problem that there is no cut-off value that could be used to diagnose oestrus in a given cow based on a single reading. Rorie *et al.* (2002) concluded that intravaginal resistance measurement was perhaps the least practical method of oestrus detection because of labour and animal handling requirements.

Table 8.2 Pregnancy rate following insemination at determined and observed oestrus. (From Ball & Jackson, 1979.)

Oestrus	No. of inseminations	No. of cows pregnant	Pregnancy rate (%)
Determined[a]	55	33	60.0
Observed[b]	132	86	65.2

[a] Cows not observed in oestrus and inseminated two and three days after milk progesterone dropped to basal levels.
[b] Cows observed in oestrus and inseminated at the normal time.

Detection of ovarian changes

Ball & Jackson (1979) monitored individual cow milk progesterone levels thrice weekly, increasing to a daily frequency five days before expected ovulation. In cows that were not observed in oestrus, insemination was carried out two and three days after progesterone readings had fallen to basal levels. The resulting pregnancy rates were not significantly different from those of other cows inseminated at observed oestrus, as is shown in Table 8.2.

Subsequent work by Foulkes *et al.* (1982) showed that this approach was practical using the more recently available enzyme-linked immunoassays for progesterone. Further developments demonstrated the feasibility of using on-farm progesterone kits in conjunction with the protocol. McLeod *et al.* (1991) devised a protocol of infrequent but strategically timed sampling for progesterone analysis in order to predict the optimum time for insemination. This has been incorporated into a commercially available computer program forming part of a fertility management package (Williams & Esslemont, 1993). The system, known as MOIRA (Management of Insemination by Routine Analysis), instructs the stockperson when to sample and, on the basis of progesterone levels measured, when to inseminate the appropriate cows. Two of the major possibilities offered by milk progesterone testing are (1) the prevention of inappropriate inseminations (see below) and (2) the detection of non pregnancy, while at the same time suggesting when to re-inseminate (see Chapter 11). On some farms, the development of automatic in-line progesterone measurement of individual cow milk progesterone levels (see Chapter 13) will offer the opportunity to take advantage of these benefits without the current high labour requirements. Progesterone measurement is the only technique that could conceivably offer an acceptable substitute for careful oestrus detection by diligent stockpeople.

'False' oestrus (oestrus not accompanied by ovulation)

It is well established that cows are sometimes recorded in oestrus at abnormal times, such as when they are pregnant or have abnormal ovarian cysts.

Observation, aided by information from progesterone profiles, suggests that recorded oestrous events not associated with normal ovulations fall into three categories:

(1)   Genuine oestrous symptoms associated with a problem such as cystic follicles.
(2)   Genuine oestrous symptoms in the absence of problems (e.g., oestrus during pregnancy). This may be caused by fluctuating levels of oestradiol produced by follicles of mid-cycle and pregnancy.
(3)   Stockperson error, including misidentification of cows.

In the second two categories, progesterone levels will in most instances remain high during the supposed oestrus. Currently available on-farm progesterone kits mean that levels can be checked before insemination is carried out, especially in cases where there is even the slightest doubt that the cow is really not pregnant and is about to ovulate.

Careful regard to the points made in this chapter, not forgetting the value of diligent record keeping and clear identification, can help to overcome the problems of false oestrus.

Summary

The only definitive behavioural sign of oestrus is that the cow will stand to be mounted by other cows or the bull. Use of a scoring system based on secondary oestrous signs offers the possibility of including many cows that might otherwise have been missed although, potentially, the timing of AI could be slightly less precise. Currently available aids to oestrus detection are not alternatives to careful and frequent observation, backed up by good records and clear identification. The only potential alternative to this is fixed-timed insemination following the artificial induction of ovulation or after the detection of a drop in milk progesterone. The measurement of a high level of progesterone can also serve to prevent the insemination of a cow that is not genuinely in oestrous. This can be especially vital if the cow is already pregnant (see Chapter 11). The reader is also referred to the comprehensive review of oestrous behaviour and its detection by Stevenson (2000).

References

Asdell, S.A. (1964) *Patterns of Mammalian Reproduction.* Cornell University Press, Ithaca, New York.

Ball, P.J.H. & Jackson, N.W. (1979) *British Veterinary Journal*, **135**, 537.

Ball, P.J.H., Morant, S.V. & Cant, E.J. (1978) *Journal of Agricultural Science, Cambridge*, **91**, 593.

Ball, P.J.H., Cowpe, J.E.D. & Harker, D.B. (1983) *Veterinary Record*, **112**, 147.

Ducker, M.J., Haggett, R.A., Fisher, W., Bloomfield, G.A. & Morant, S.V. (1983) *Animal Production*, **36**, 519.

Fordham, D. (1984) *Oestrus detection in dairy cows by milk temperature measurement.* PhD thesis, University of Newcastle.

Foulkes, J.A., Cookson, A.D. & Sauer, M.J. (1982) *British Veterinary Journal*, **138**, 515.

Heckman, G.S., Foote, R.H., Oltenacu, E.A.B., Scott, N.R. & Marshall, R.A. (1979) *Journal of Dairy Science*, **62**, 64.

Kiddy, C.A. (1977) *Journal of Dairy Science*, **60**, 235.

Kiddy, C.A., Mitchell, D.S., Bolt, D.J. & Hawk, H.W. (1978) *Biology of Reproduction*, **19**, 389.

Lyimo, Z.C., Nielen, M., Ouweltjes, W., Kruip, T.A. & van Eerdenburg, F.J. (2000) *Theriogenology*, **53**, 1783–1795.

Maatje, K., Loeffler, S.H. & Engel, B. (1997) *Journal of Dairy Science*, **80**, 1098–1105.

McLeod, B.J., Foulkes, J.A., Williams, M.E. & Weller, R.F. (1991) *Animal Production*, **52**, 1–9.

MLC (1983) *Beef Yearbook*.

MMB (1982) *Breeding & Production*, **32**.

Mottram, T.T.F. & Frost, A.R. (1997) *Silsoe Research Institute Report*.

Rorie, R.W., Bilby, T.R. & Lester, T.D. (2002) *Theriogenology*, **57**, 137–148.

Stevenson, J.S. (2000) In *Fertility in the High Producing Cow* (ed M.G. Diskin). *British Society of Animal Science Occasional Publication*, **26**, 43–62.

Stevenson, J.S., Smith, M.W., Jaeger, J.R., Corah, L.R. & LeFever, D.G. (1996) *Journal of Animal Science*, **74**, 729–735.

Van Eerdenburg, F.J., Loeffler, H.S. & van Vliet, J.H. (1996) *Veterinary Quarterly*, **18**, 52–54.

Van Eerdenburg, F.J., Karthaus, D., Taverne, M.A., Merics, I. & Szenci, O. (2002) *Journal of Dairy Science*, **85**, 1150–1156.

Williams, M.E. & Esslemont, R.J. (1993) *Veterinary Record*, **132**, 503–506.

Chapter 9
Artificial Control of the Oestrous Cycle

An understanding of the hormones that control ovulation in the natural cycle has enabled the development of procedures that use exogenous hormone treatments to control oestrus and ovulation for the benefit and convenience of the cattle breeder. Such treatments may be used either in individual animals or in groups to synchronize ovulation. Reproductive physiologists and veterinarians have sought reliable systems of control of the oestrous cycle for many years, since they would offer several management advantages:

- Successful methods of oestrous cycle control would facilitate the use of artificial insemination (AI) thereby allowing the greater exploitation of genetically superior sires. At present AI is underutilized particularly in beef cattle.
- AI could be carried out at a prearranged or fixed time if the control method was sufficiently reliable. This could potentially remove the need for the detection of oestrus. However, as will be seen later, the optimum performance is achieved when control of the cycle is used in conjunction with oestrus detection. In fact it may be said that control of the cycle serves to improve the rate of oestrus detection by concentrating the occurrence of induced heats into a shorter finite period of time.
- Synchronization of oestrus would allow the batch management of inseminations and calvings which in some circumstances would improve the efficiency of management. This is particularly true in groups of replacement heifers and in beef suckler cows, which are usually managed in groups and do not always receive the frequent and individual attention accorded to dairy cows. Under traditional conditions heifers and suckler cows are served naturally, due in part to the practical difficulties associated with the detection of oestrus. Therefore the use of pharmacological agents to control the oestrous cycle could potentially increase the use of AI in these situations.
- Synchronization may offer some advantages in shortening the calving to conception interval, and thus the calving interval and possibly the calving season, particularly in beef herds. The importance of these parameters in determining reproductive efficiency is discussed in Chapter 1.

There are, however, a number of real or potential disadvantages to synchronization of ovulation:

- Currently, response to treatment and subsequent fertility are highly variable. Results vary considerably between herds and between years in the same herd. Consequently, the economic factors are variable also, but if reproductive performance is poor there will obviously be a low or negative cost benefit.
- There are often unseen costs such as the necessity for an increased labour input as compared to a natural mating system, in that the cows have to be collected and handled more frequently.
- Inseminators may tire and become less efficient if too many animals are to be served on one day.
- Adverse factors on any one day can affect a large number of animals' ability to conceive, rather than just one or two.
- If successful, synchronization of a large batch of animals may result in excessive demands on labour and facilities at and just after calving

Principles and methods of cycle control

The control of the oestrous cycle is dependent on manipulation of hormonal changes in order to cause ovulation at a predetermined, convenient time, rather than when it would have occurred naturally. There are three main approaches:

- The artificial induction of premature luteolysis using luteolytic agents such as prostaglandin $F_{2\alpha}$ ($PGF_{2\alpha}$). This will obviously only be effective in cycling cows with an active corpus luteum.
- Prostaglandin-induced luteolysis in association with GnRH to manipulate follicular and luteal function. This procedure could potentially be used for the induction of ovulation in acyclic as well as cyclic cows.
- The simulation of corpus luteum function, by administration of progesterone (or one of its synthetic derivatives) for a number of days, followed by abrupt withdrawal. This procedure is also effective for the induction of ovulation in acyclic cows.

The artificial induction of premature luteolysis

The most potent luteolytic agents available are derivatives of $PGF_{2\alpha}$. Injection of exogenous $PGF_{2\alpha}$ or one of its analogues during the mid-luteal phase of the cycle results in premature luteolysis and a consequential fall in peripheral progesterone concentrations. This is followed by a rise in secretion of gonadotrophins and oestradiol-17β, culminating in the pre-ovulatory surges and eventual ovulation. The fall in progesterone concentrations is rapid, invariably reaching basal levels within 30 hours of injection (Fig. 9.1).

The time of ovulation after the injection can be quite variable, depending on whether there happens to be a dominant follicle present at the time of luteolysis. This will depend on the stage of the cycle and whether the cow is

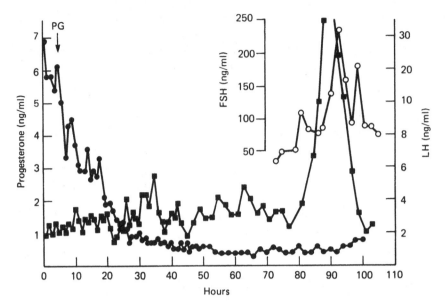

Fig. 9.1   Plasma concentrations of progesterone (●), LH (■) and FSH (○) in a cow after injection of tiaprost (an analogue of PGF$_{2\alpha}$). Note the decrease in progesterone concentrations and LH and FSH pre-ovulatory surges after 80–90 hours.

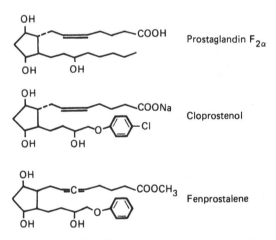

Fig. 9.2   Molecular structure of PGF$_{2\alpha}$ and some analogues.

undergoing a two- or three-wave cycle (see Chapter 4). The molecular structure of PGF$_{2\alpha}$ and some of its analogues, which are available commercially for oestrus synchronization, is shown in Fig. 9.2.

Prostaglandins have been used to control the oestrous cycle in several different ways. Some possible methods are:

- Following rectal examination so that only those cows with a corpus luteum are injected. These cows should then show oestrus and ovulate 3–5 days later. This method has the disadvantage that it is time-consuming and that rectal palpation involves added expense. The results also depend on the accuracy of the rectal palpation.
- Following the identification of an active corpus luteum using milk progesterone measurement. A further milk sample could be taken before intended AI in order to confirm that the prostaglandin injection had induced luteolysis.
- Observation of all cattle for oestrus for a seven-day period, serving any that show oestrus. The rest are injected with prostaglandin on the following day and may be inseminated either once or twice at fixed times or at observed oestrus. The reason for the initial seven-day observation period is that there is a period of about seven days in the cycle (day 18 to day 0 and day 1 to day 4) when the animal is unresponsive to prostaglandin, i.e. when no corpus luteum is present. After seven days, those originally between days 18 and 0 should have shown heat and been served, while those that were between days 1 and 4 will now be between days 8 and 11, i.e. in the mid-luteal phase, and therefore responsive to prostaglandin.
- The two injection plus two insemination method. The so-called two plus two technique was designed to synchronize groups of animals cycling at random without prior knowledge of their precise ovarian status. All cattle are injected on day 1 of treatment and the injection repeated 11 days later. AI is then carried out usually three and four days later. Alternatively, cows may be served at observed oestrus after the second injection. At the time of the first injection some animals will be responsive to the prostaglandin, i.e. between days 5 and 17 of the cycle. These will undergo luteolysis in response to the injection and will ovulate some four days or so later. At the time of the second injection (11 days later) these cows will be on about day 8 of the next cycle. The cows that were not responsive to the first injection, i.e. those between days 18 and 4 of the cycle, would be between days 8 and 15 at the time of the second injection. Therefore all animals are theoretically in the responsive mid-luteal phase at the time of the second injection. The technique is popular and quite successful in synchronizing cycles in heifers. However, pregnancy rates in lactating cows have not always been consistent and reasons for this are discussed later. The principle of this regimen is illustrated in Fig. 9.3.
- A modification of the 'two plus two' method is the so-called 1½ method. Cows are injected with prostaglandin and those that show oestrus are inseminated. Those that have not been seen in oestrus are injected again 11 days after the first injection and may be inseminated either at a fixed time(s) or at observed oestrus. Although requiring further effort in terms of oestrus detection, this method tends to give better results than the 'two plus two' regime and is perhaps the current method of choice. Its main advantage, however, is the reduction in cost by the reduction of both the number of treatments used and number of inseminations per cow.

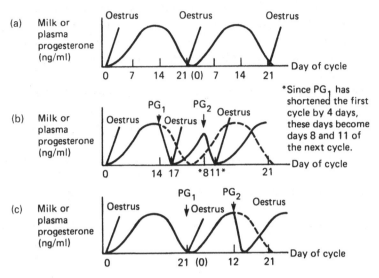

Fig. 9.3 Principle of the 'two plus two' method of prostaglandin usage. (a) Changes in progesterone concentrations during two natural oestrous cycles. (b) Effect of giving the first prostaglandin injection during the luteal phase, e.g. on day 14. (c) Effect of giving the first prostalandin injection during the follicular phase, i.e. on day 21. Solid line indicates actual progesterone profile; dashed line indicates progesterone profile if no treatment given. (After Peters, 1984.)

- The use of GnRH in conjunction with prostaglandin. The so-called Ovsynch regimen (Pursley *et al.*, 1997) was designed to reduce the variability in the time of ovulation following the use of prostaglandin alone. GnRH is injected on day 0, followed by prostaglandin on day 7 and a further GnRH injection on day 9–10. Fixed-time AI is performed 16 hours later. The first GnRH injection is designed to either (1) manipulate ovarian follicular development by ovulating and/or luteinizing the existing dominant follicle and initiating the growth of a new cohort of follicles so that a new dominant follicle emerges by day 7, or (2) extend the life of the existing corpus luteum in late-luteal phase cows so that it is still responsive to prostaglandin 7 days later. The second GnRH injection is designed to synchronize ovulation further by initiating the pre-ovulatory LH surge, which should initiate ovulation. Peters *et al.* (1999a,b) found that 'Ovsynch', with the second GnRH being given on day 9.5, was effective and suggested that the major role of the first injection appeared to be the extension of the cycle in late-luteal phase cows and that the second GnRH injection was the most critical in determining the synchrony of ovulation.

The simulation of corpus luteum function using progesterone

In this method the function of the corpus luteum is simulated by the administration of progesterone or one of its derivatives. The progesterone suppresses gonadotrophin release, and hence follicular maturation, until it is withdrawn. If a group of cows is treated with progesterone and then it is withdrawn from all cows simultaneously, this will theoretically synchronize ovulation in the group. In order to synchronize a group of randomly cycling cows effectively, it is necessary to treat them with progesterone for a period equivalent to the length of the natural luteal phase, i.e. at least 16 days. This is due to the fact that exogenous progesterone has little or no effect on the life span of the natural corpus luteum and therefore in some cases the natural corpus luteum might outlive a short-term progesterone treatment, resulting in a failure of synchrony. However, it has been shown that long-term progesterone treatments (18–21 days) result in poor pregnancy rates (Fig. 9.4). This is due at least in part to the ovulation of persistent follicles that ovulate oocytes of reduced fertility and possibly also to adverse changes in the intra-uterine environment, which inhibit sperm transport.

Shorter-term progesterone treatments (7–12 days) generally result in more acceptable pregnancy rates (Fig. 9.4), but unfortunately tend not to control the cycle adequately since, if treatment is started early in the cycle, the natural corpus luteum may outlast the progesterone treatment. Therefore it is necessary to incorporate a luteolytic agent with short-term progesterone treatments in order to eliminate any natural corpus luteum. For this reason, oestradiol

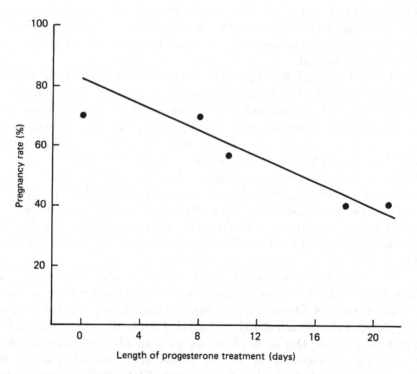

Fig. 9.4 Effect of length of exogenous progesterone treatment on pregnancy rate in heifers following insemination at the induced oestrus. (Adapted from Roche, 1974.)

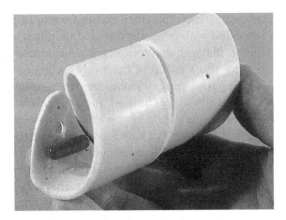

Fig. 9.5 A progesterone-releasing intravaginal device (PRID).

and/or a luteolysin is used in combination with short-term (7–12 days) progesterone treatments.

Implants are the most suitable method of administration of progestogens
since withdrawal can then be precisely controlled by implant removal. They can
be inserted into the vagina or under the skin, usually in the ear. Products for
insertion in the vagina include the progesterone-releasing intravaginal device
(PRID; Sanofi Ltd.), which consists of a stainless-steel coil covered by a layer
of grey inert silastic (Fig. 9.5) in which 1.55 mg progesterone is impregnated. A
red gelatin capsule containing 10 mg oestradiol benzoate is attached to the
inner surface of the coil.

The PRID is inserted into the vagina by means of a speculum and is left in
place for up to 12 days. The oestradiol benzoate in the gelatin capsule is rapidly
absorbed through the vaginal wall into the systemic circulation and is intended
to act as a luteolytic agent. The progesterone is released continuously from the
elastomer until removal of the device. Removal is effected by pulling on the
string which is left protruding from the vulva after coil insertion.

PRID contains natural progesterone and therefore its effects can be
monitored by measuring progesterone concentrations in the blood plasma
or milk of the animal. Fig. 9.6 shows the effects on the ovarian cycle of
administering progesterone, e.g. PRID, under different conditions. PRID treatment can also be effective in acyclic cows (see Chapter 12). This is illustrated
in Fig. 9.7.

A less bulky alternative (which could thus potentially be preferable for
heifers) is the bovine controlled internal drug releaser (CIDRb; DEC-InterAg)
as shown in Fig. 9.8. Originally, an oestradiol capsule was incorporated for
luteolysis, but an intra-muscular (i.m.) injection on the day of insertion is now
the preferred option. Day *et al.* (2000) reported an advantage from using an
i.m. injection of oestradiol on the day of insertion (instead of a capsule)
and a further oestradiol injection 48 hours after CIDR withdrawal to control

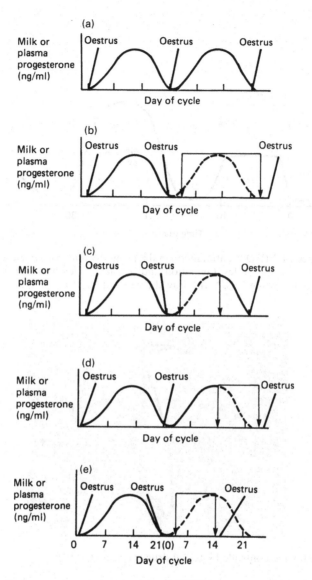

Fig. 9.6 Effect of progesterone treatment, e.g. PRID, on progesterone concentrations when administered under various conditions. (a) Two natural cycles. (b) 21-day progesterone treatment starting on day 4. (c) 10-day progesterone treatment starting on day 4. (d) 10-day progesterone treatment starting on day 14. (e) Luteolytic agent given with a 10-day progesterone treatment starting on day 4. Solid line indicates actual progesterone profile; dashed line indicates progesterone profile if no treatment given. (After Peters, 1984.)

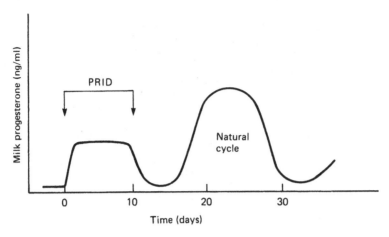

Fig. 9.7 Effect of PRID treatment on milk progesterone concentrations in a cow not undergoing ovarian cycles. Ovulation and ovarian cycles may also be induced in non-cyclic cows following PRID withdrawal (see Chapter 10).

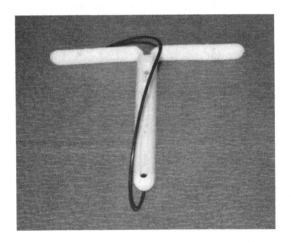

Fig. 9.8 The bovine controlled internal drug releaser (CIDRb).

follicular development. This should increase the precision of oestrus onset and the intensity of oestrous signs as well as more tightly controlling the timing of the LH surge and thus ovulation, so that the timing of AI can be optimized (Diskin *et al.*, 2000). Luteolysis by means of an injection of prostaglandin the day before CIDR removal has also proved effective (e.g., Lucy *et al.*, 2001).

The other approach is to use an impregnated silastic subcutaneous implant (Crestar; Synchromate B; Intervet). The active ingredient is Norgestomet (17α-acetoxy-11β-methyl-19-nor-preg-4-ene,20-dione), a synthetic analogue of progesterone. The implant is inserted subcutaneously behind the ear for a period of nine days during which time the progesterone is absorbed into the blood circulation. The implant is removed by making a small scalpel incision in the skin of the ear over the implant. At the time of the implantation an intra-muscular injection of 5 mg oestradiol valerate is given as a luteolysin, in combination with an initial injection of 3 mg Norgestomet. Removal of the device after 7–12 days causes peripheral plasma progesterone concentrations to fall, thus simulating natural luteolysis. Consequently, the cow should show oestrus 48–72 hours later and fixed-time AI may be used at these times. This product is suitable for use in heifers so that there is no problem of withdrawing milk from sale during treatment.

Dealing with cows that are not pregnant after synchronization regimes

Once synchronized cows have been inseminated, it is important to detect those that are not pregnant as early as possible and to take appropriate action. The simplest approach is to observe cows for oestrus and to re-inseminate them if and when this is observed. This can be labour intensive and detection efficiency may be poor – two possible reasons for choosing to synchronize in the first place!

It may be appropriate to resynchronize non-pregnant animals. This may be particularly so in the case of heifers, but has also been shown to be successful in lactating cows. Eddy (1983) gave two injections of cloprostenol at an interval of 11 days to all cows, followed by AI at 72 and 96 hours after the second injection. Twenty-four days after the second AI, milk samples were taken for progesterone assay (see Chapter 8). Cows diagnosed not pregnant were given a further dose of cloprostenol seven days later (31 days after the second AI) and inseminated again at 72 and 96 hours. Pregnancy was checked by rectal palpation about seven weeks after the first insemination, negatives again being injected with cloprostenol. In this way fertility indices of the herd improved dramatically within one year, e.g. the conception rate increased by 10%, the calving to conception interval was reduced by almost 20 days and a benefit to cost ratio of 3.5:1 was calculated. Stevenson *et al.* (2003) scanned dairy cows for pregnancy diagnosis 27–29 days after first service at fixed-time AI, assuming that a first-wave dominant follicle was present at that time. This would be expected to ovulate in response to GnRH after luteolysis with prostaglandin. Insemination at observed oestrus after prostaglandin alone or at fixed time after prostaglandin followed by GnRH both significantly reduced calving to conception intervals as compared to non-pregnant cows that were not treated but served on the basis of observed oestrus alone.

Factors affecting pregnancy rate after the controlled ovulation

It cannot be overemphasized that in order to maximize results obtained with pharmacological control of the oestrous cycle, nutritional status and general management must be of a high standard. As discussed in Chapter 7, the major limiting nutritional factor in reproduction is probably energy intake, as crudely assessed by body weight or, preferably, body condition score. Recommended body condition targets for cows in various reproductive states are specified in Chapter 14 and these should be given particular attention when cycle control is used.

Physiological problems in cycle control

The efficacy of the pharmacological control of ovulation can be considered as two components:

- The degree of synchrony following treatment. That is, the proportion of animals beginning to show oestrus or ovulating within a specified time period after the end of hormonal treatment.
- Subsequent reproductive performance (e.g., pregnancy rate), which will also to an extent be dependent on the degree of synchrony, particularly if fixed-time AI is used.

Synchrony following treatment

In view of the variation in timing of the behavioural and ovarian events around natural oestrous periods (Table 4.2), it is perhaps not surprising that even after hormone treatment there is still considerable variation in the timing of responses between animals. Hence where fixed-time AI is used, two inseminations are usually incorporated into many of the protocols described in order to maximize the probability of conception. Regimens using more than one hormone tend to be more effective in this regard, to the extent that only one rather than two fixed-time inseminations may be acceptable. This must be balanced against the increased labour and drug costs.

In some cases, there may be a lack of synchronization as a result of a failure of complete luteolysis, which has occurred in 10% or more of cows treated with prostaglandins. It takes the form of either a complete lack of effect on progesterone concentrations or, for example, a fall to 50% of pre-injection levels, followed by luteal recovery usually within 24–48 hours. Causes of luteolytic failure are not clear but may be related to several factors including treatment too early in the luteal phase and non-responsiveness of some corpora lutea even in the appropriate phase of the cycle. Some of the more complex regimens were designed to overcome this. Other reasons include incorrect injection site or technique (e.g., injections that should be intramuscular may be injected accidentally into fat or ligamentous tissue) and a short half-life of the exogenous prostaglandin in the animal.

In up to 20% of cows injected with prostaglandin, although luteolysis appears to occur normally, progesterone concentrations remain low for an unusually long period and this may be associated with an abnormally long delay until oestrus and ovulation. This partly depends, as we have said, on whether there happens to be a dominant follicle present at the time of luteolysis, and again the more complex regimens such as 'Ovsynch' were designed to rectify the problem. It must be remembered that extended follicular phases (>8 days) also occur in about 17% of untreated dairy cows (P.J.H. Ball, unpublished data). Thus it is likely that this phenomenon is related at least in part to an aberration in the adult cow's ovarian cycle and may well be related to the effects of nutritional and other stresses as discussed in Chapter 12. The problem has not been reported in heifers and certainly the cycles of adult cows would appear to be less uniform than those of heifers.

The ovary can only respond to prostaglandin if there is a functional corpus luteum. Therefore cows not undergoing activity do not respond. The proportion of cows in this state will vary from herd to herd and with the average stage post-partum, but it is generally regarded as a more serious problem in suckling beef cows (see Chapter 7). For this reason it is recommended by some pharmaceutical companies that prostaglandins are not used before day 42 after calving. Progestagen and GnRH-based treatments may be more appropriate in this regard, but the underlying reasons for ovarian activity should also be considered.

Failure of synchrony after progestogens may occur if the associated luteolytic agent is ineffective (prostaglandins may be preferred over oestradiol in this respect) or if there is a failure to maintain high blood concentrations of progesterone, resulting in the occurrence of oestrus and ovulation before removal of the device. This premature fall has occurred particularly with the intravaginal method of administration, probably as a result of progesterone-induced changes in absorption across the vaginal wall rather than exhaustion of progesterone in the device. The problem can be best avoided by minimizing the length of the treatment period. However, it is inadvisable to reduce the length of treatment below seven days, since this would result in inadequate synchronization.

Field-scale evaluation of oestrus synchronization techniques

Many field trials have been carried out to assess the effect of the various treatments on reproductive performance. These will not be discussed in detail here, but they may be summarized as follows:

- In adult cows conception rates after synchronization have varied widely as compared to control cows served at naturally occurring oestrus, and there has been a tendency for them to be worse. If fixed-time AI is used, the timing may not be sufficiently precise.
- Fertility results are often up to 20% better in heifers than in cows.
- In general, single fixed-time AI might be expected to result in 10–15% lower pregnancy rates than two fixed-time AIs. Some results have challenged this

Table 9.1   Effect of cloprostenol treatment of cyclic cows which had not been observed in oestrus by day 50 postpartum. (From Ball, 1982.)

Treatment	Time of insemination	No. of cows	Calving to conception interval (days)
None until 90 days after calving	Observed oestrus	166	107.4
Cloprostenol[a]	Observed oestrus	61	98.1
Cloprostenol[a]	2 and 3 days after injection	75	104.0

[a] 0.5 mg cloprostenol (Mallinckrodt) was injected intramuscularly 10–14 days after ovulation had occurred as judged from three-times weekly milk progesterone measurements.

assumption, and the choice will depend to an extent on the regimen used for synchronization.

• It is clear that best reproductive performance is achieved when oestrous cycle control is combined with insemination at observed oestrus. This would be expected to improve the timing of AI and in that situation the reproductive performance of treated cows may often be higher than that of controls. This may happen particularly in a herd where the efficiency of oestrus detection is normally low. Following a synchronization treatment, it is expected that the vast majority of cows would show oestrus within ten days after treatment. Therefore, the effect of treatment in this situation is to concentrate the occurrence of oestrous periods, so that detection efficiency can be increased over a relatively short time. Results of a study of use of the prostaglandin analogue cloprostenol with either fixed-time AI or observed oestrus are shown in Table 9.1 and illustrate the advantage of insemination at observed oestrus.

Summary

A number of different approaches to the artificial control of the cow's oestrous cycle have been described. Their use may be limited according to individual country regulations concerning, e.g., the ability to sell milk after treatment with a particular hormone. Generally speaking, recent protocols involving more than one hormone tend to be more effective but also more costly and time consuming.

It is difficult to be precise about the cost–benefits of oestrus synchronization since these may vary from region to region, with the regimen used, with the effectiveness of the treatment and the reproductive efficiency of the herd before treatment. In any case, any estimate made is soon overtaken by inflation. For a comprehensive review of oestrus synchronization see Diskin *et al.* (2000).

References

Ball, P.J.H. (1982) *British Veterinary Journal*, **138**, 546.

Day, M.L., Burke, C.R., Taufa, V.K., Day, A.M. & Macmillan, K.L. (2000) *Journal of Animal Science*, **78**, 523–529.

Diskin, M.G., Sreenan, J.M. & Roche, J.F. (2000) *British Society of Animal Science Occasional Publication*, **26**, 175–193.

Eddy, R.G. (1983) *British Veterinary Journal*, **139**, 104.

Lucy, M.C., Billings, H.J., Butler, W.R., Ehnis, L.R., Fields, M.J., Kesler, D.J., Kinder, J.E, Mattos, R.C., Short, R.E., Thatcher, W.W., Wettemann, R.P., Yelich, J.V. & Hafs, H.D. (2001) *Journal of Animal Science*, **79**, 982–995.

Peters, A.R. (1984) *Veterinary Record*, **115**, 164.

Peters, A.R., Mawhinney, I., Drew, S.B., Ward, S.J., Warren, M.J. & Gordon, P.J. (1999a) *Veterinary Record*, **145**, 516–521.

Peters, A.R., Ward, S.J., Warren, M.J., Gordon, P.J., Mann, G.E. & Webb, R. (1999b) *Veterinary Record*, **144**, 343–346.

Pursley, J.R., Kosorok, M.R. & Wiltbank, M.C. (1997) *Journal of Dairy Science*, **80**, 301–306.

Roche, J.F. (1974) *Journal of Reproduction and Fertility*, **40**, 433.

Stevenson, J.S., Cartmill, J.A., Hensley, B.A. & El-Zarkouny, S.Z. (2003) *Theriogenology*, **60**, 475–478.

Chapter 10
Artificial Insemination

Introduction: the advantages of artificial insemination

Artificial insemination (AI) has many advantages to offer the dairy farmer, but problems of oestrus detection limit the value of AI in beef herds. Some of the most important advantages of AI, as opposed to natural service, are outlined below:

- genetic gain
- cost effectiveness
- disease control
- safety
- flexibility
- fertility management.

Genetic gain

This is probably the major advantage of AI and, together with disease control, was one of the main reasons for its development. The technique enables superior genes to be spread widely amongst the cattle population. Individual farmers have access to genetic material from bulls that can be carefully tested, following selection from a large population of available stock. The costs of such a selection and testing programme, which would be prohibitive to an individual, can thus be shared between the users of the AI service.

A danger in using a single bull to inseminate all the cows in a herd is that he may be carrying a genetic defect that is only manifested in his offspring – perhaps not until they are mature – by which time the damage will have been done. The chances of such a defect remaining hidden after the testing of AI bulls before their semen is offered for sale are small. On the other hand, if the defect occurs at a low frequency, so that it is not detected during progeny testing, the affected bull could be used for many thousands of inseminations before the problem is found. The problem could thus cause more damage to the cattle population as a whole. It was recently discovered that the recessive gene causing bovine leucocyte auto-immune deficiency (BLAD) – similar to human HIV and usually leading to the death of heterozygous recessive calves – was present in a bull widely used for AI. Fortunately, a test is now available to detect the problem gene so that this particular problem can be eliminated. On balance, the genetic advantages far outweigh the potential risks.

Cost effectiveness

Even if a herdsperson is not interested in the potential gains from using genetically superior stock available through AI, he/she may still find that the economic advantages make the use of the service worthwhile. A bull can be expensive to buy or rear, and there is always the risk of the bull proving unsatisfactory and having to be disposed of prematurely. Furthermore, it may not be discovered that a bull is infertile or subfertile until he has been with a group of cows for some months. By this time, the herd's calving pattern will have been severely disrupted, adding to the financial losses. Once the bull is in use it will still cost its owner money to maintain an otherwise unproductive animal, and under most circumstances that money would be better spent on another cow to produce a saleable product.

Disease control

If a bull is infected with a venereal disease not only may this render him infertile, but also he may infect any cow that he serves. Trichomoniasis and campylobacteriosis, for example, can be spread in this way. The Welsh AI centres were set up specifically to control these diseases. Other diseases, such as brucellosis, while not strictly venereal, can still be spread by means of physical contact between the bull and the cows he serves. If a bull is shared with, or hired out to, other farms, the risk of spreading infection is obvious.

The precautions taken in the course of providing an AI service make it very unlikely that infection could be spread by this means, and the use of AI has contributed to a significant reduction in the incidence of venereal diseases. In the UK, for example, trichomoniasis has been brought under control as a result of the development of AI.

It must be said that, if an infectious agent can survive the precautions taken, there is the risk of a more widespread dissemination of infection through the medium of AI. Semen imports to the UK from the USA were banned for many years in case the bluetongue virus should enter the country in imported semen. As with genetic gain, the advantages of AI in preventing the spread of infection heavily outweigh the potential risks.

Safety

Some people feel that the safety aspect of keeping a bull was one of the major stimuli to the setting up of AI services. Any bull is potentially dangerous, but this varies to some extent between breeds. A Hereford bull, for instance, is much less liable to be aggressive than a Friesian or a Holstein. However quiet a bull may appear, there is always the possibility that he will become aggressive. In many cases this factor alone will tip the balance in favour of using AI.

Flexibility

A herd manager may not wish all calves to be sired by bulls with the same characteristics, or even of the same breed. He or she may wish to breed the best milkers to a good dairy bull, and to use a beef bull on low-yielding or problem cows and on maiden heifers of dubious potential. When breeding his or her best cows in the hope of obtaining good replacements the herd manager may use bulls with certain characteristics that complement those of the particular cow. If, for example, a cow produces milk in large quantities but with a low fat content, the herd manager may decide to use a bull with a good record for fat production; on another cow with high fat production but with bad udder conformation he or she may use a bull known for the good udder conformation of his daughters. It is impracticable to keep enough bulls to cover all possible requirements, and AI is the obvious answer.

Fertility management

By using AI, the time of each insemination can be controlled and recorded. By knowing the time of a successful insemination, the time to dry-off, for example, can be predicted. With natural service, this is usually only possible through the practice of hand mating, which is very labour intensive.

The history of AI

The earliest recorded use of AI was as long ago as 1780 in Italy when a bitch was induced to produce pups by this method. It was not until around 1900 that serious attempts were made to develop the technique in farm animals. The work was carried out by Ivanov and colleagues in Russia, and by 1930 they had achieved success with cattle and sheep. Within the next ten years AI was in commercial use for cattle in the USA and the UK. The first AI centre in the UK was established at Cambridge. This was followed by the Ministry of Agriculture, Fisheries and Food's Cattle Breeding Centre, which operated near Reading, and its centre in North Wales, which was subsequently sold to the Milk Marketing Board of England and Wales (MMB). The MMB undertook the creation of a national AI service in 1944 with the takeover of an independent AI centre. The creation of another 23 centres by 1951 meant that the MMB, together with a small number of independent organizations, was providing an AI network that covered the whole of England and Wales. Similar progress was being made in North America, with the development of large commercial AI corporations and cooperatives.

The development by Polge and co-workers at Cambridge in 1949 of a method of freezing semen ranks with the discovery of penicillin in that it had far-reaching consequences and resulted, at least in part, from an accident. Apparently the labels on two bottles inadvertently became swapped. The crucial factor was the discovery that glycerol could be used to protect bovine spermatozoa from damage during freezing. Within three years the technique had undergone field trials and semen frozen by means of solid carbon dioxide was available commercially. By 1963 the use of liquid nitrogen for even lower temperature storage was being evaluated. This meant that, with careful handling, semen could be stored for very long periods of time. Frozen semen was originally stored in glass ampoules, or sometimes as pellets. A refinement in frozen semen storage – the plastic straw – was invented in Belgium and developed in France. The MMB brought 0.25-ml plastic straws into general use for the freezing and handling of semen in 1973.

These developments have resulted in well over half of the dairy cattle in England and Wales being bred by AI. The figure is similar for most European countries, and somewhat less than 50% in the USA. Almost all the dairy cattle in Denmark and Japan are bred by AI. On 31 January 2002 the Milk Marketing Boards in the UK were dissolved because they were not consistent with European Community legislation. The MMB's commercial arm, Genus, still provides an AI service, but a number of other companies do so as well, so that national statistics for AI usage are no longer available. In the meantime, there has been an increase in the practice of 'do-it-yourself' AI (DIYAI). The serious outbreak of foot-and-mouth disease in the UK in 2001 prevented AI technicians from visiting farms and subsequently led to an increase in applications for DIYAI training.

AI in developing countries

In developing countries limitations of technology and communications have restricted the development of AI services. In Pakistan, for example, the service is limited to the close vicinity of the AI stations because when the cattle come into oestrus they have to be brought in to the stations by their owners. Communal grazing of cattle in many countries, such as Zimbabwe, makes it very difficult to ensure that the appropriate cow is inseminated artificially and not by a neighbour's bull. Problems of distance and terrain are often compounded by the smallness of herds, as in parts of Colombia, adding to the difficulties of oestrus detection. However, in a small herd, the economic disadvantages and potential problems of keeping a bull are proportionately greater, and means of facilitating the introduction of AI should be encouraged. In parts of Ethiopia and Indonesia, where some herds are very small, good progress has been made in developing a technician-based AI service. Technology from developed countries, such as cow-side progesterone tests, may well be worthy of consideration in some of these situations.

Sire selection

The procedures used by commercial organizations, such as Genus, Semex and Cogent, to select and evaluate Friesian, Friesian × Holstein and Holstein sires for their AI studs are illustrative of the effort that goes into the selection and evaluation of a good AI sire. Details can be found in Chapter 15.

Semen collection

Routine semen collection from a dairy bull begins after he has proved himself in the selection procedures described in Chapter 15. By this time he is likely to be around six years of age. Beef bulls usually start to produce semen for commercial use from under two to about three years of age.

Most semen collections are carried out by inducing the bull to ejaculate into an artificial vagina. This is constructed to simulate the feel of a cow's vagina. Water at about 45°C is held between the casing and a synthetic rubber sleeve. This helps to provide the right sensation for the bulls, some of which have very precise preferences in this regard. The artificial vagina incorporates a synthetic rubber cone to channel the semen into a test tube for collection. Insulation around the test tube protects it from damage and keeps the semen just below body temperature until it reaches the laboratory for further processing. A freshly prepared, sterile artificial vagina is used for each collection. The details of a typical artificial vagina are shown in Fig. 10.1. It is usual to collect semen from a bull as it mounts a suitably restrained live teaser animal such as a steer, another bull or a cow (Fig. 10.2). Bulls can also be trained to mount an artificially constructed dummy. This system was developed in France and is used routinely there and elsewhere.

The quality and quantity of semen produced is enhanced by 'teasing' the bulls before they are collected. This usually involves encouraging them to indulge in one or more 'false' mounts before they are given the opportunity to ejaculate. Sometimes the teaser animal may be changed between mounts.

If a bull's semen is collected too frequently the volume and quality produced at each ejaculation will be reduced. In practice, there has to be a compromise

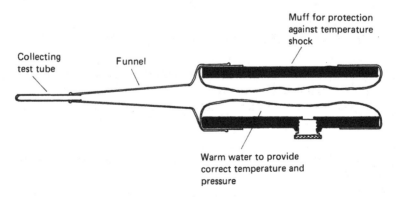

Fig. 10.1   An artificial vagina for collection of bull semen.

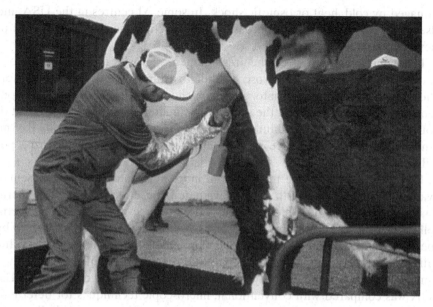

Fig. 10.2 Semen collection using a live teaser. (Courtesy of Genus.)

between maximum total production and a reasonable yield at each collection. This means that most bulls are collected about twice a week throughout their productive life, which usually lasts for 5–6 years.

Semen evaluation

Once semen has been collected it is maintained at a temperature of 30–35°C until it has been evaluated and is ready for further processing.

An initial assessment of the quality of the semen can be made immediately after collection. If it appears fairly clear the concentration of spermatozoa will be unacceptably low. If the semen is not of reasonably uniform consistency or contains pus the presence of infection is indicated. The semen should also be checked visually at this stage for the presence of contaminants such as hair, faeces or blood. The presence of urine can also be detected at this stage. The volume of semen in an ejaculate can also be measured by means of graduations on the test tube immediately after collection. Low volume in itself gives no cause for worry, since there is considerable variation between individuals and between collections. Semen volume may also be reduced as the result of frequent collection.

A small sample of the semen is placed on a slide on a warm (30°C) microscope stage in order to estimate the proportion of live spermatozoa. At least 60% of the spermatozoa should be swimming with a normal wave motion. If spermatozoa are swimming backwards or in circles they could well have been damaged by cold, heat or osmotic shock. In some AI centres in the USA and elsewhere, examination is made easier by projecting the microscope field of view onto a television screen.

Following examination of the fresh semen, nigrosin stain is added to a diluted semen sample on a microscope slide to estimate the proportion of morphologically abnormal spermatozoa, which should not exceed 20%. The concentration of spermatozoa in the semen is estimated from the measurement of optical density of a sample diluted in buffered formal saline (normally 0.05 ml semen in 10 ml saline). There should be at least 500×10^6 spermatozoa per millilitre of semen.

Efforts have been made to develop a more automated process for semen evaluation. Palmer & Barth (2003) evaluated the effectiveness of a sperm quality analyser (SQA), which contains a densitometer for determining sperm cell concentration and an optical sensor to evaluate light deflections caused by sperm movement. Analysis of light deflections enables the generation of a value called the sperm quality index (SQI). The SQI represents the quality of a semen sample defined by sperm motility, concentration, viability and morphology. The SQA was compared with conventional, microscopic techniques for determining the percentage of motile sperm and sperm concentration in bull semen samples and evaluated for its ability to classify bulls as satisfactory or unsatisfactory potential breeders. The results suggested that it was not a reliable substitute for conventional semen analysis and was not useful for determining bull breeding soundness.

Freezing, storage and distribution of semen

Almost all of the semen used in AI in developed countries is frozen to preserve it during storage and distribution. This is most successfully achieved if the semen is stored in liquid nitrogen at a temperature of −196°C. Before freezing the semen is diluted in a suitable extender. This contains ingredients appropriate to its functions, which are:

- dilution
- protection against cold shock
- cryoprotection
- energy source
- buffering
- maintenance of osmotic pressure
- inhibition of bacteria.

Dilution

A diluent is required to act as a carrier for the other components of the extender and so that individual doses of semen are of a volume that is convenient to handle and store. Most of the semen now used for AI is handled in plastic straws of 0.25-ml capacity, although 0.5-ml straws are still available. A typical ejaculate of around 8 ml may contain 10×10^9 spermatozoa. This is sufficient for 500 units of 20×10^6 spermatozoa. In order to obtain units of 0.25 ml as required, the ejaculated semen needs to be diluted around 15 times. The constituents of the extender are made up in double-distilled water or UHT milk to the required dilutions. Obviously, overdilution can adversely affect conception rates and semen companies will aim for a dilution rate that will maximize economic return, while not compromising fertility. Garner *et al.* (2001) reported that the addition of seminal plasma could be used to attenuate the dilution effect.

Protection against cold shock

In the absence of protective agents, sperm cells would be cold-shocked as semen was cooled significantly below body temperature. Egg yolk (usually around 10% by volume) is commonly used to minimize this. Milk, or a combination of egg yolk and milk, may also be used. Foote *et al.* (2002) reported that constituents of milk also acted as anti-oxidants, protecting sperm against reactive oxygen species that may be present during processing before freezing. They suggested that additional anti-oxidants might be beneficial in egg-yolk-based extenders, as was confirmed by Bilodeau *et al.* (2002), who reported that the addition of low amounts of catalase and millimolar concentrations of pyruvate greatly improved the antioxidant properties of a commonly used extender.

There have been attempts to move away from animal-based cryoprotectants, which may pose hygienic risks and are difficult to standardize. There has also been a suggestion that cows that fail to conceive to a given insemination may develop immunity to the protein in the egg or milk, and thus be more difficult to breed at a subsequent insemination. A new generation of semen diluents free of animal ingredients is available. A sterile soybean extract is often used instead of egg yolk or milk. Thun *et al.* (2002) compared such an extender with a conventional egg yolk Tris extender and found that the latter generally gave better fertility, but that results varied between breeds. However, Aires *et al.* (2003) reported clear benefits from using a soy lecithin extender as compared to an egg-yolk-containing extender.

Cryoprotection

Unprotected sperm cells are ruptured and killed as ice crystals form during the course of freezing. As has been said, the discovery that glycerol provided protection for sperm during freezing had dramatic effects on the practicality of AI. When egg yolk is used, just less than 7% by volume of glycerol is added after initial cooling of the semen to 5°C.

Energy source

Spermatozoa need a source of energy if they are to survive in vitro. This is normally supplied by means of a simple sugar such as fructose.

Buffering

Lactic acid is produced as an end product of sperm metabolism. This can cause a harmful lowering of pH. Citrate, phosphate and Tris buffers are commonly used to overcome this, although they are not necessary when a lactose diluent is used. For some reason the use of Tris as a buffer has the advantage that there is no need to wait until after initial cooling to add the glycerol.

Maintenance of osmotic pressure

The concentration of constituents, such as sugars, in the extender must be such as to avoid its being hypo-osmotic in relation to the spermatozoa, which could otherwise be ruptured.

Inhibition of bacteria

Addition of antibiotics serves to control bacteria, such as those responsible for vibriosis. Extenders should always be made up fresh, under clean conditions. In spite of these precautions it is still possible that viral diseases, such as bluetongue, may be transmitted in semen used for AI. Cattle in the UK are free of this disease, but it is a problem in some countries, including parts of Europe, the USA and Australia. It is thus necessary to restrict the movement of semen between certain countries.

Constituents used in typical commercially available diluents are shown in Table 10.1.

At present, all of the semen used for AI in the UK is frozen, stored and distributed in plastic straws, which are labelled and filled by specially designed machines. Once the straws have been filled, they are cooled to 5°C and then allowed to equilibrate before freezing. The straws are then brought down to −110 to −130°C at a controlled rate. Cooling too fast can cause thermal shock and cooling too slowly can result in increased osmotic pressure as water freezes out. This can cause irreparable damage to the spermatozoa. Computer-controlled machines are now available to control the temperature drop automatically. The straws are stored in liquid nitrogen at −196°C in large insulated vacuum flasks. Semen straws and the equipment for handling and storing them are illustrated in Fig. 10.3.

As an alternative to straws, a system of microencapsulation of bovine spermatozoa has been developed. Polymer membranes are used to form capsules ranging in diameter from 0.75–1.5mm (Nebel *et al.*, 1993). The process could

Table 10.1 A common formulation for a Tris-based extender for bovine semen.

Function	Constituent	Quantity	
Buffer {	Tris buffer[a]	24.24 g	} Supplied as a concentrate
	Citric acid	14.00 g	
Energy source	Fructose	10.00 g	
Cryoprotectant	Glycerol[b]	50 ml	
Diluent	Purified water[c]	800 ml	
Cold shock protection	Egg yolk	200 ml	
Antibiotic[d]			

[a] Also known as Sigma 7–9.

[b] This gives a glycerol concentration of 6.25% in a single-step dilution. For a two-step dilution, semen is diluted to half the final volume in glycerol-free extender. The dilution is completed after chilling, using extender with 12.5% glycerol.

[c] The concentrate is dissolved by boiling in approx 750 ml purified water. On cooling, the volume is adjusted to 800 ml with purified water and the pH adjusted to 6.7 before adding the egg yolk.

[d] Antibiotics are required by law to be added to the extender. The EU Directive 88/407 specifies 500 µg streptomycin, 500 iu penicillin, 150 µg lincomycin and 300 µg spectinomycin per ml or 'an alternative combination of antibiotics with an equivalent effect against campylobacters, leptospires and mycoplasmas'.

be of value when small quantities of semen are used, as may be available following semen sexing procedures.

A new technique has been developed which optimizes ice crystal morphology during the freezing of sperm cells and thus minimizes damage from ice crystals at thawing (Arav *et al.*, 2002). The toxic effect of glycerol is also reduced, since less is required. Semen is frozen in a 'multi thermal gradient' freezing apparatus, which moves the container at a constant velocity through a thermal gradient, producing a controlled cooling rate.

Insemination

DIY vs technician service

Do-it-yourself AI offers a number of potential advantages over a technician service, but there may be disadvantages as well (see Table 10.2). On average, similar results should be obtained for DIY and for the technician service. Some operators may do better, and others may do worse! Where possible, the farmer should keep open the option of calling in a technician in special circumstances.

As with the commercial technician service, DIY is subject to regulations that cover aspects such as disease transmission and animal welfare. In the UK, a licence for an on-farm tank can only be obtained when one or more people from that farm have satisfactorily completed an approved course, such as is run by Semex UK. Such certificated personnel may only inseminate cows on the licensed premises. New regulations are currently being formulated by the UK Department for the Environment, Food and Rural Affairs.

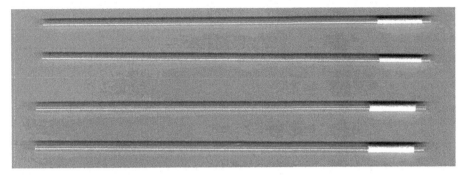

(a)

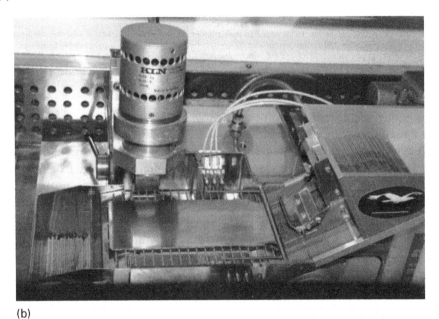

(b)

Fig. 10.3 Equipment for handling and storage of semen. (a) Plastic straws designed for storage and handling of a single dose of semen. (b) Straws being filled with semen. (c) Semen freezing. (d) Straws stored in flasks of liquid nitrogen. (Courtesy of Genus.)

Insemination procedures

For conception to occur, insemination must take place at the correct stage of the cow's oestrous cycle. Bovine spermatozoa require a few hours in the female reproductive tract to capacitate and become capable of fertilization and they remain viable for about 24 hours. The egg is most likely to become fertilized if it contacts viable spermatozoa within about 6 hours of ovulation, and has a maximum life of about 12 hours. Thus the timing of AI must be fairly precise. The optimum time to inseminate is 12–24 hours after the beginning of

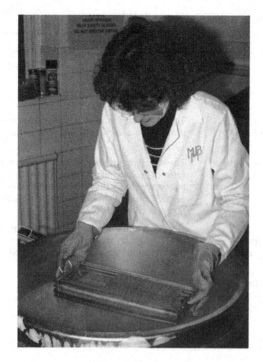

(c)

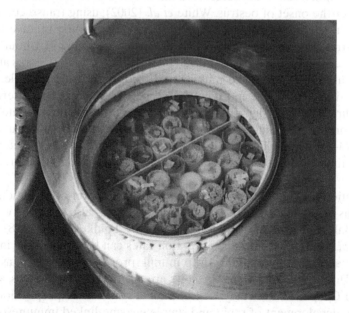

(d)

Fig. 10.3 *Continued.*

Table 10.2   The advantages and disadvantages of DIYAI.

Advantages of DIYAI	Advantages of technician service
The insemination can be carried out at the optimum time, and it is simpler to carry out a repeat insemination if oestrus is prolonged	The technician is likely to be a highly trained professional
The cow should not need to wait in isolation and/or in strange surroundings until the technician arrives	The technician is likely to be getting more practice on a variety of different cows
The operator has a personal interest in the cow and the result	The AI company should check the non-return rates of technicians and retrain them as necessary (but with DIY an accurate record of performance should be kept and action taken in case of problems)
The cow should be used to the inseminator, whereas she may be upset by the presence of a stranger – especially one that looks like a vet!	If there is only one inseminator on the farm, a day off or an off day could cause inseminations to be missed or botched
There should be cost savings once the semen tank and other equipment are paid for	

standing oestrus (see Saacke *et al.*, 2000). This ensures that sperm arrive at the site of fertilization a few hours before ovulation, which normally occurs around 30 hours after the onset of oestrus. White *et al.* (2002), using transrectal ultrasonography in beef cows, reported that the time of ovulation relative to the onset of oestrus was constant during all seasons and averaged 31.1 hours.

In practice, good timing is best achieved by watching cows for oestrus at least three times a day in addition to milking and feeding times. If possible, cows first observed in heat in the morning should be inseminated that afternoon, and those first showing signs in the afternoon should be inseminated the following morning. Saumande (2001) called this advice into question, but in the absence of 24-hour surveillance by farm staff or electronic devices to determine the precise time of onset of standing oestrus, the traditional advice remains the best.

Insemination can also be carried out after the induction of ovulation with progestogens or luteolytic agents (see Chapter 9). It was also shown in work at Reading (Ball & Jackson, 1979) followed up by Foulkes *et al.* (1982) and McLeod *et al.* (1991) that normal conception rates can be obtained by inseminating cows at a fixed time after a drop in milk progesterone levels has been measured. This is true even when the cows are not observed in oestrus, as was discussed in Chapter 8. This may well become a commercial proposition as a result of the development of rapid and simple enzyme-linked immunosorbent assay (ELISA) techniques for milk progesterone measurements. It would be particularly useful in conjunction with automatic, in-line progesterone measurement at milking (see Chapter 13).

The cow to be inseminated must be in oestrus without any doubt and should be properly prepared for the insemination. While awaiting service, she should be in a good holding area in familiar surroundings with (if waiting for more than about 15 minutes) adequate fresh water and a ration of the food that she would normally be eating. To reduce the stress of isolation from the herd, it may be worth keeping her 'oestrus playmate' with her until it is time to inseminate. In any case, the waiting time should be kept to an absolute minimum.

The insemination facilities should be clean, airy and well lit. The AI stall should restrain the cow comfortably, but tightly, so that she cannot move backwards, forwards or from side to side. A good crush may be suitable, but she should be used to entering it routinely and not just when she is going to get injected or foot trimmed! The cow should be at the right height for the inseminator. A stable step should be provided if necessary. There should be a suitable shelf or table for equipment, and the necessary gloves, paper towels, warm disinfected water, etc. should be in place before removing the straw of semen from the liquid nitrogen.

Semen in the farm tank or inseminator's portable tank or flask must remain frozen and immersed in liquid nitrogen until the moment it is removed from storage for immediate use. Even if the semen does not actually thaw, if the temperature is allowed to rise irreparable damage occurs on recooling to liquid nitrogen temperature. The rate of thawing should be controlled, and this will vary according to the pattern of temperature fall during freezing. The usual procedure is to immerse the straws in water at 35°C for 20–30 seconds when using 0.25-ml straws or 40–60 seconds for 0.5-ml straws. Thawing kits are available for this purpose.

The sealed end of the straw is then removed with sharp scissors and the straw loaded into a specially made 'gun' (Fig. 10.4), being secured in place by a clean, new, disposable plastic sheath. A further disposable plastic sleeve ('chamise sanitaire') is recommended to protect the gun from contamination as it is passed through the vagina.

It is important to use each dose of semen promptly after it has been thawed. Kaproth *et al.* (2002) reported that there was no fall in conception rate for up to 20 minutes after thawing when a highly competent technician performed the insemination, but in practice an absolute maximum of 15 minutes should be aimed for. It is vital that the semen is not allowed to cool after it has been

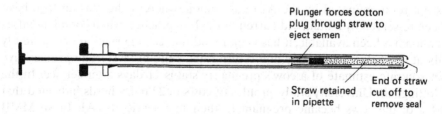

Plunger forces cotton plug through straw to eject semen

Straw retained in pipette

End of straw cut off to remove seal

Fig. 10.4   Insemination gun.

thawed. The straw in the insemination gun should be insulated, especially in cold weather. It has been suggested that insemination should be carried out without first thawing the semen. This would mean it would thaw inside the cow and that there was no opportunity for recooling. More investigation is needed before this procedure can be recommended.

The semen is introduced straight from the straw into the cow's tract. With the cow suitably restrained, the AI technician grasps the cervix per rectum, pulls it towards him, and holds it level so that the insemination gun can be introduced through the vagina into the cervical os. If a 'chamise sanitaire' is used, the end of the gun is pushed through the end of the sleeve just before the gun is passed into the cervix. The tip of the pipette is passed just through the cervix so that semen is injected into the uterine body. The aim is to ensure that the end of the pipette is absolutely in line with the anterior end of the cervix, but does not go through it at the time of semen injection. If the pipette is inserted too far, all of the semen may end up in one uterine horn. In the USA and elsewhere it is normally recommended that cows are inseminated just into the uterus at their first service, but that at repeat services semen is deposited in the cervix. This very sensible precaution avoids insertion of the pipette into the uterus, which could well cause abortion should the cow happen to be pregnant to a previous service. The practice is not followed in the UK because, supposedly, there is a reduced chance of conception if the cow is not already pregnant. In fact, conception rates are only likely to be reduced by about 5% if the gun is more than half way through the cervix. The use of a milk progesterone test to avoid wrongly timed inseminations would remove the need for such a decision.

Dalton *et al.* (2000) have reviewed the factors affecting pregnancy rates following insemination.

The success of AI

Given the high standards attained by AI organizations, the technique should give a conception rate equivalent to that obtained using natural service. In spite of the widespread use of AI (well over 50 million inseminations have been carried out in England and Wales alone), surprisingly few accurate data are available on actual conception rates. Most of the available data are based on non-return rates. This means that a cow will be assumed to be pregnant if she is not re-inseminated by the AI organization, whereas she may, in fact, have been re-served by a bull, sold barren or died. In practice, when complete information has been available, it has been found that calving rates are consistently about 8% below 90/120-day non-return rates. Milk progesterone profiles give an accurate estimate of a cow's pregnancy status 21 days after service. In the Nottingham University study, profiles of cows in 22 dairy herds indicated that 64% of the cows became pregnant to their first service by AI. In an MMB survey (T.R.B. Lewis, unpublished information), AI and natural service were used in approximately equal proportions in each of 12 pedigree Friesian herds involving 1059 cows and heifers. The average live calving rates to first AI and first natural insemination were almost identical at 64.05% and 64.5%, respectively. The non-return rate for artificially inseminated cows as calculated from AI centre records was approximately 12% higher than the calving rate.

References

Aires, V.A., Hinsch, K.D., Mueller-Schloesser, F., Bogner, K., Mueller-Schloesser, S. & Hinsch, E. (2003) *Theriogenology*, **60**, 269–279.

Arav, A., Zeron, Y., Shturman, H. & Gacitua, H. (2002) *Reproduction Nutrition Development*, **42**, 583–586.

Ball, P.J.H. & Jackson, N.W. (1979) *British Veterinary Journal*, **135**, 537.

Bilodeau, J.F., Blanchette, S., Cormier, N. & Sirard, M.A. (2002) *Theriogenology*, **57**, 1105–1122.

Dalton, J.C., Nadir, J., Bame, M., Noftsinger, M. & Saacke, R.G. (2000) *British Society of Animal Science Occasional Publication*, **26**, 175–193.

Foote, R.H., Brockett, C.C. & Kaproth, M.T. (2002) *Animal Reproduction Science*, **71**, 13–23.

Foulkes, J.A., Cookson, A.D. & Sauer, M.J. (1982) *Veterinary Record*, **111**, 302.

Garner, D.L., Thomas, C.A., Gravance, C.G., Marshall, C.E., DeJarnette, J.M. & Allen, C.H. (2001) *Theriogenology*, **56**, 31–40.

Kaproth, M.T., Parks, J.E., Grambo, G.C., Rycroft, H.E., Hertl, J.A. and Gröhn, Y.T. (2002) *Theriogenology*, **57**, 909–921.

McLeod, B.J., Foulkes, J.A., Williams, M.E. & Weller, R.F. (1991) *Animal Production*, **52**, 1–9.

Nebel, R.L., Vishwanath, R., McMillan, W.H. & Saacke, R.G. (1993) *Reproduction Fertility and Development*, **5**, 701–712.

Palmer, C.W. & Barth, A.D. (2003) *Animal Reproduction Science*, **77**, 173–185.

Saacke, R.G., Dalton, J.C., Nadir, S., Nebel, R.L. & Bame, J.J. (2000) *Animal Reproduction Science*, **60–61**, 663–677.

Saumande, J. (2001) *Revue de Medecine Veterinaire*, **152**, 755–764.

Thun, R., Hurtado, M. & Janett, F. (2002) *Theriogenology*, **57**, 1087–1094.

White, F.J., Wettemann, R.P., Looper, M.L., Prado, T.M. & Morgan, G.L. (2002) *Journal of Animal Science*, **80**, 3053–3059.

Chapter 11
Pregnancy Diagnosis

The accurate diagnosis of pregnancy is of crucial importance in the establishment and maintenance of optimal reproductive performance. It is desirable for the farmer to know as soon as possible if a mated cow is not pregnant, so that she can be rebred with the minimum delay. Until fairly recently pregnancy diagnosis consisted of observation for oestrus, especially at about 21 days after service. Given that oestrus detection efficiency and accuracy are low in most herds (see Chapter 8), reliance on this method results in a large number of non-pregnant cows assumed to be pregnant and some pregnant cows being inseminated inappropriately, which could abort them (see Chapter 12). Furthermore, a large number of cows sold as barren are found, at slaughter, to have been pregnant.

A number of other methods have been developed over the years, and there follows a description of potentially useful methods and suggestions for their optimal use in cattle fertility management.

Methods of pregnancy diagnosis

Non-return to service

Traditionally, a cow was diagnosed as non-pregnant if she was seen in oestrus (and, as a rule, re-inseminated) approximately 21 days after service. The percentage of cows not seen in oestrus at about this time is known as the non-return rate and is an established method of estimating pregnancy rates. It is usually the first method (in terms of time after service) used by the stockperson to discriminate between non-pregnant and pregnant cows.

Since the percentage of ovulating cows actually seen in oestrus is often as low as 50% (see Chapter 8), the non-return rate usually overestimates pregnancy rates and, in the individual cow, can easily lead to a false sense of security. However, an effective procedure for detecting oestrus in non-pregnant cows is still a very important aspect of good reproductive management. It is useful to have a recording system which will draw attention to cows due to return, but, of course, this should not be to the detriment of observation at other times in case of returns at abnormal intervals.

If a cow is recorded in oestrus approximately three weeks after service, it is still possible that she could be pregnant. Inseminating her is very likely to cause abortion. Great care should be taken to confirm that she is genuinely in heat and not pregnant. A 'cow-side' milk progesterone test (see below) could be used and insemination avoided unless the progesterone level is very low. If insemination is carried out and there is any possibility of an existing pregnancy, then the AI pipette should not be passed all the way through the cervix (see Chapter 12 in section 'Insemination during pregnancy'). Oestrous behaviour and oestrus detection are discussed in Chapter 8.

Progesterone measurement

The detection of pregnancy by measurement of hormones, particularly if they occur in milk, has an advantage over rectal palpation in that interference with the cow is minimal and there is a negligible risk to the pregnancy. The measurement of progesterone to check for pregnancy also offers the possibility of diagnosis at day 21 or even earlier.

Progesterone is secreted by the corpus luteum throughout pregnancy. As was discussed in Chapter 5, peak values are usually reached by about day 10 after ovulation and are subsequently maintained, whereas in the non-pregnant animal levels fall at about day 17 of the cycle. Consequently, in the pregnant cow, blood and milk progesterone concentrations remain high between days 21 and 24 after ovulation, when they would be basal in the non-pregnant animal (see Fig. 5.5). Therefore a sample taken at this time may be used to discriminate between the pregnant and non-pregnant cow. The development of rapid highly sensitive ELISA (enzyme-linked immunosorbent assay) procedures has allowed the commercial exploitation of this test. The introduction of monoclonal, rather than polyclonal, antibodies (Groves *et al.*, 1990) lowered the limits of detection and increased the discrimination of the assays.

The simplest procedure is to take a milk sample from the cow at about 20 days after insemination. If the progesterone level is low, the cow is definitely not pregnant, provided that the right sample has been taken from the correct cow and the test has worked properly. If the progesterone level is high, the cow could be pregnant (Fig. 11.1).

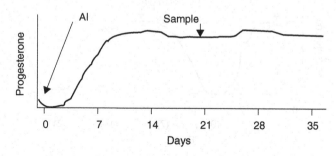

Fig. 11.1 Schematic representation of correct positive milk progesterone pregnancy diagnosis.

The exact day to sample could range from 19 (when a low progesterone value would signal a careful watch for oestrus, enabling a prompt return service) to 24 (giving the cow a chance to show heat on return, so that there would be no need to sample). It is important to obtain a bulk milk sample since the progesterone concentration is dependent on the level of milk fat, which is in low concentration in foremilk and high concentration in strippings. This is of obvious importance if the method is used for beef suckler cows since the time of sampling in relation to the calf suckling can affect the result. The test could also be carried out after blood sampling in non-lactating animals such as maiden heifers. This may stress the animal and would involve veterinary intervention and its associated costs.

The concentration of progesterone reflects the function of the corpus luteum, but not necessarily the presence of an embryo or fetus. A high progesterone level suggests that the cow is pregnant, but a single test like this is only about 80% accurate for positive pregnancy diagnoses. There are a number of reasons for false positive tests:

- The cow may not be pregnant but the life of the corpus luteum may still be extended for some reason, such as a uterine infection (see Chapter 12).
- The cow could have been inseminated at the incorrect stage of the cycle, i.e., during the luteal phase. At the time of the test, she is likely to be in the luteal phase of the subsequent cycle, and the progesterone level would be high. (Fig. 11.2) A sample taken at the time of AI would help to confirm that the timing was right and improve the accuracy of the pregnancy diagnosis sample (Fig. 11.3).
- The diagnosis may be accurate, but the embryo or fetus is lost afterwards (Fig. 11.4). This is now quite common – see Chapter 12. A further sample 42 days after AI may fail to show that this has occurred since ovarian cycles may have been re-established, making it likely that a high progesterone level would be measured on the day of the subsequent sample (Fig. 11.5).

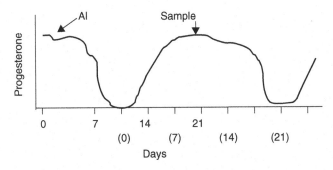

Fig. 11.2 Schematic representation of false positive milk progesterone pregnancy diagnosis in a cow inseminated at the wrong time.

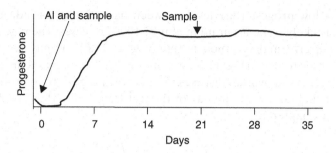

Fig. 11.3 Schematic representation of correct positive milk progesterone pregnancy diagnosis.

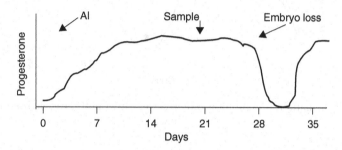

Fig. 11.4 Schematic representation of correct positive milk progesterone pregnancy diagnosis, but in a cow that subsequently lost her conceptus.

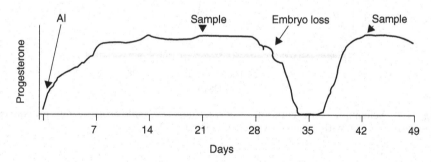

Fig. 11.5 Schematic representation of milk progesterone pregnancy diagnosis in which a second sample failed to reveal an embryo loss.

- Other reproductive problems, such as luteinized cystic follicles, could lead to high progesterone levels on the day of the pregnancy diagnosis test.

In summary, approximately 80–85% of positive diagnoses between days 21 and 24 appear to be accurate, i.e., they result in a calf being born at the appropriate time. Therefore 15–20% of cows with high progesterone levels at days 21–24 do not calve subsequently, i.e., they are false positives. In contrast, the finding of a low progesterone level between days 21 and 24 indicating non-pregnancy is likely to be accurate in almost 100% of cases. The cow may have failed to conceive and returned normally (Fig. 11.6) or may have inactive ovaries, or cystic follicles (Fig. 11.7), so that no progesterone is being produced. Other types of cystic ovarian disease cause erratic progesterone production, so that levels could be low on the day of the test (Fig. 11.8). These problems are described in Chapter 12.

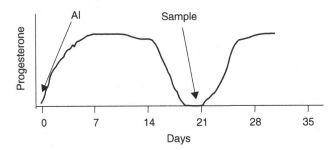

Fig. 11.6   Schematic representation of correct negative milk progesterone pregnancy diagnosis.

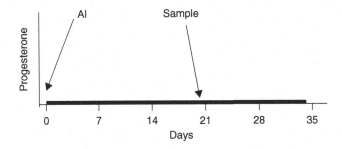

Fig. 11.7   Schematic representation of correct negative milk progesterone pregnancy diagnosis in a cow with inactive ovaries or cystic follicles.

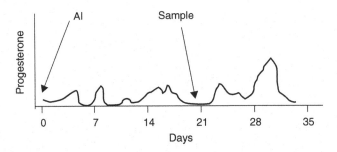

Fig. 11.8   Schematic representation of correct negative milk progesterone pregnancy diagnosis in a cow with luteinized cystic follicles.

In any event, a low progesterone level in a correctly sampled and tested milk sample means that the cow will certainly not be pregnant. Thus, milk progesterone measurement may be considered as a highly accurate test for non-pregnancy and can be very useful in allowing early rebreeding, providing cycles are normal. In fact, as was shown in Chapter 8, it is possible to use a series of milk samples taken from about day 18 after insemination not only to detect pregnancy failure, but also to determine the time to re-inseminate, even if oestrus is not observed.

Milk progesterone pregnancy testing was first applied in the UK by the Milk Marketing Board in the mid 1970s. A single bulk milk sample was taken between days 21 and 24 after insemination and despatched to the laboratory by post for assay. The associated delay in receiving results tended to cancel out the advantages of testing early after insemination. The development of a test that could be carried out on farm (commonly known as the 'cow-side test') enabled results to be obtained rapidly and thus be of more potential use in reproductive management. A number of 'cow-side' progesterone test kits are now available, offering the possibility of results within hours, or even minutes, of sampling at very cost effective prices. However, it is currently estimated that less than 5% of dairy cows in Great Britain are tested using the milk progesterone method. The development of an automated assay to measure individual cow progesterone levels at milking is eagerly awaited by many farmers with large herds and computerized milking parlours. The development of such assays is discussed in Chapter 13.

As was seen in Chapter 5, cows with lower progesterone levels as soon as day 5 after insemination are likely to have lower pregnancy rates (Table 5.2). Marshall *et al.* (2003) found that milk progesterone levels on day 6 after insemination were almost twice as high in cows subsequently diagnosed pregnant as in those diagnosed non-pregnant. Even so, individual variation within both pregnant and non-pregnant cows means that there is little chance of using this measurement as a very early diagnostic test. They also measured an increase in milk progesterone levels from day 5–6 of 3 ng/ml in subsequently pregnant cows compared to 1 ng/ml in non-pregnant cows and suggest that, if the results were repeated with larger numbers of cows, this could be a possible means of making a tentative, but potentially useful, very early diagnosis of pregnancy.

Pregnancy-specific proteins

Early pregnancy factor (EPF) is a pregnancy-dependent protein complex that has been detected in the serum of several species (Morton *et al.*, 1983). It is detected using an immunological technique, the rosette inhibition test. It is claimed that this substance appears in serum shortly after conception and disappears very rapidly following embryonic death. Therefore the detection of EPF would offer a very valuable method of pregnancy diagnosis. Whilst a degree of success has been achieved using this technique in some laboratories (e.g., Yoshioka *et al.*, 1995), results in the cow have been insufficiently reproducible to offer much immediate hope of an improved method of pregnancy diagnosis.

Two further proteins, bovine pregnancy-specific protein B (bPSPB) and bovine pregnancy associated glycoprotein (bPAG – an antigen synthesized in the superficial layers of the ruminant trophoblast), can be measured during early pregnancy in the cow with much more reliability. Szenci *et al.* (1998b) found that the use of either of these proteins compared favourably with ultrasound pregnancy at days 26–58 after AI, although the accuracy of detecting non-pregnant animals by both protein tests was limited by the relatively long half-life of these proteins after calving and by early embryonic mortality. They reported significantly fewer false positive diagnoses by the bPSPB test than by the bPAG test.

Patel *et al.* (1997) reported that peripheral bPAG concentrations in Holstein cows after non-surgical embryo transfer were correlated to the stage of gestation and fetal number, and that the profile of the peripheral plasma concentrations provided a useful indication of feto-placental status. Humblot (2001) has reviewed the use of pregnancy-specific proteins to monitor pregnancy and study late embryo mortality in ruminants.

bPAG has been produced commercially but is currently not available in the UK. The main drawbacks to its routine use in pregnancy diagnosis are that it is only detectable in blood and not milk, plus the carryover from the previous pregnancy and the failure of levels to fall promptly after conceptus loss (e.g., Szenci *et al.*, 1998a).

Real-time ultrasound scanning

The availability of real-time β-mode ultrasound scanning has been a major advance in pregnancy diagnosis and reproductive monitoring in a number of species including man, sheep, dogs, horses and cattle. It has the advantage that it is non-invasive apart from the requirement in the large farm species for insertion of a rectal transducer, and thus it is a very safe procedure. Pregnancy can be detected as early as 17 days using this method.

A very comprehensive account of the use of ultrasound to examine the bovine reproductive tract is given by Boyd (1991), but a brief summary of the detectable changes in early pregnancy is worthwhile here. The conceptus begins to occupy the contralateral horn by about day 17 after service and it can be observed as a non-echogenic (dark) area. By day 19 the amniotic sac has expanded considerably and therefore the lumen of the uterus can readily be observed. By day 22 it is possible to see the beating embryonic heart and by day 30 the conceptus is so obvious that a very rapid and accurate diagnosis can be made. By day 35 the uterine caruncles can be visualized individually. Later, fetal age can be determined approximately by the measurement of crown rump length. A series of ultrasound images of various stages of pregnancy is shown in Fig. 11.9.

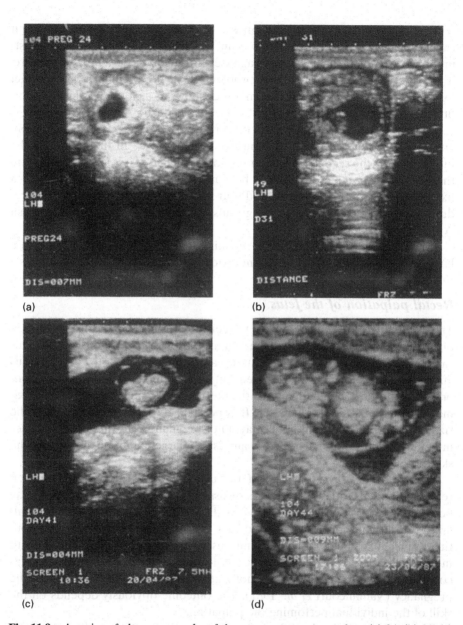

Fig. 11.9 A series of ultrasonographs of the pregnant uterus on days (a) 24, (b) 31, (c) 41 and (d) 44. The uterine lumen can be seen clearly as an anechoic (dark) area and the developing embryo as an echogenic (lighter) structure inside the lumen, increasing in size and definition with age. The placental membranes are clearly visible in sections (c) and (d) and the limb buds in (d) (day 44). (Reproduced by kind permission of Prof. J.S. Boyd and Drs S.N. Omran and N. Mowa.)

This method of pregnancy diagnosis has a double advantage in that it can be carried out relatively early – in practice from about 28 days post-insemination – and that positive diagnoses are highly accurate. Furthermore, it is sometimes possible to detect problems with the pregnancy and predict losses. For example, an infection sometimes shows as a cloudiness in the amniotic fluid, which would normally give a clear black echo.

If the scan is carried out between four and five weeks after insemination, any cow or heifer that failed to conceive is likely to be in the middle of the luteal phase of the second cycle after insemination and, if it is absolutely certain that she is not pregnant, she could be synchronized with prostaglandin for a fixed-time re-insemination three and four days later. We have used the procedure successfully in synchronized groups of maiden heifers at the Scottish Agricultural College (SAC).

It has been suggested that early scanning may actually cause loss, but in a large-scale study at SAC we found no evidence of this.

Rectal palpation of the fetus

This technique relies on the ability to feel the presence of a fetus swelling in one of the uterine horns by inserting an arm into the rectum of the cow. This can be a hazardous process since trauma can be inflicted on both cow and fetus and should therefore only be carried out by a trained operator. In the non-pregnant and early pregnant animal the uterine horns can be felt to be approximately equal in size and diameter. It is possible to detect a difference in the size of the two horns from about day 40 of pregnancy onwards. This is easier in heifers than in multiparous cows and is to a large extent dependent on the skill of the operator.

If, from about day 30, a fold of the uterine wall is picked up and then released, the sensation of two layers of tissue passing through the fingers may be felt. This so-called membrane-slip is due to the presence of the chorioallantois inside the horn. It is advised that this technique is not practised routinely, since it has been known in some cases to damage the fetus and to result in fetal death and abortion. However, following a survey of 7500 cows, it was concluded that this technique did not significantly affect the outcome of the pregnancy (Vaillancourt *et al.*, 1981). The outcome obviously depends on the skill of the individual performing the palpation.

From 6–8 weeks the disparity in horn size becomes quite marked, the pregnant horn becoming up to six times the diameter of the non-gravid horn at 10 weeks. After this stage the non-gravid horn also begins to enlarge due to the invasion and attachment of the placenta throughout the uterine lumen. By 12 weeks the diameter of the pregnant horn may be 10 cm or more and is easily detectable (see Fig. 11.10).

As the gravid uterus becomes larger and heavier it begins to sink down below the pelvic brim and by the fifth month it may not be possible to palpate it. Only when the fetus has grown further, to the seven-month stage, may it be

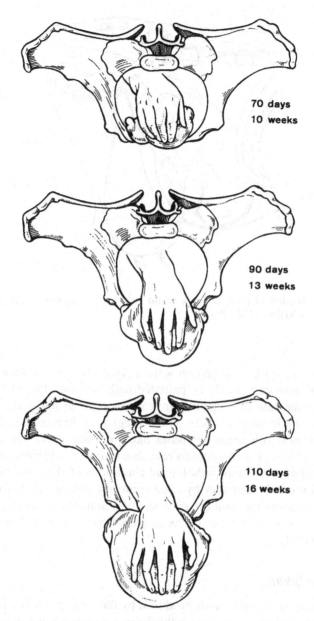

70 days
10 weeks

90 days
13 weeks

110 days
16 weeks

Fig. 11.10   Detection of pregnancy by rectal palpation. (Redrawn from Arthur *et al.*, 1982.)

possible to feel it again. However, in these cases pregnancy may be suspected by the absence of the normal reproductive tract in the pelvic cavity and the palpation of the cervix and anterior vagina as a taut band of tissue passing over the pelvic brim. The presence of cotyledons may or may not be felt from about the fourth month onwards. The sensation is quite characteristic and has been

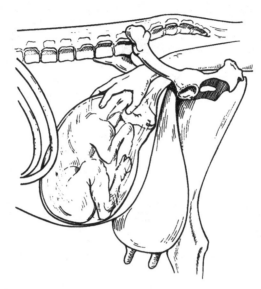

Fig. 11.11 Detection of pregnancy by rectal palpation. Pregnancy approaching term. (Redrawn from Arthur *et al.*, 1982.)

described as like 'corks bobbing on water'. After the seventh month of gestation the fetal head can usually be palpated with ease (see Fig. 11.11).

Another indication of pregnancy may develop about mid-term. Blood flow through the middle uterine artery on the pregnant side increases dramatically during pregnancy. This usually pulsates like a normal artery, but in advanced pregnancy slight compression of this reveals a characteristic vibrating sensation known as fremitus. Certain pathological conditions of the uterus can be confused with a normal pregnancy by causing uterine enlargement. These include pyometra, large tumours and the presence of a mummified fetus.

The detection of pregnancy by rectal palpation is described in more detail by Noakes (1991).

Oestrone sulphate

The identification of compounds produced by the conceptus rather than by the dam would have clear advantages in the diagnosis of pregnancy in farm animals. Oestrogens are produced by the bovine conceptus and oestrone sulphate concentrations in maternal plasma rise from about day 70 of pregnancy. The oestrone sulphate content of milk reflects that of plasma and it has been found that a positive oestrone sulphate test at 15 weeks of pregnancy gives a 100% accurate diagnosis of pregnancy. In most cases, detection of non-pregnancy at this late stage is of limited value to reproductive management, but it can be used as a confirmatory test following an earlier positive diagnosis, such as a milk progesterone test at 21–24 days. If there is any reason to suspect that a cow has aborted, the oestrone sulphate test can be very useful in determining her status.

Mammary development

Mammogenesis or development of the mammary gland occurs as a consequence of pregnancy (see Chapter 6) and in the primiparous heifer changes can be detected as early as four months of gestation. In addition, a viscous brown secretion may be expressed from the teats. Of course, these changes are not apparent in the parous, lactating cow. Steroidal-type growth promoters can elicit identical changes in the mammary glands of heifers. This can be an additional confounding factor in countries and situations where they are used. It is only during the last few days of pregnancy when the udder becomes distended with colostrum that mammary development can be regarded as an accurate diagnosis of pregnancy.

Ballottement

The abdomen of the pregnant animal begins to become distended from about seven months of gestation. If a hand is pushed firmly against the right side of the abdomen, the fetus may sometimes be felt to rebound against it. This technique is commonly used in cattle markets by prospective purchasers. However, it is not a reliable indicator of pregnancy particularly if the findings are negative.

Conclusions

A summary of available methods of pregnancy diagnosis is given in Table 11.1. Pregnancy diagnosis is a vital aid to reproduction management and the stock person should aim for the best combination of earliness and accuracy. For this reason, more than one diagnosis is recommended for each cow. As a minimum, an early milk progesterone test to achieve the earliest possible re-insemination of non-pregnant cows should be followed by a final confirmation of pregnancy, either manually or by ultrasound scan, at about 72 days, after which we consider the pregnancy to be relatively secure. Ideally, an intermediate diagnosis by ultrasound scan between days 28 and 42 should be carried out to get an early and accurate diagnosis. The cost should not be alarming when balanced against the cost of getting it wrong. The cost of the 'cow-side' progesterone test is very small when compared with the benefits, and the timing of the final diagnosis is not critical, so that larger batches of cows can be examined to reduce the cost.

It should be emphasized that pregnancy diagnosis is of little use without a planned programme for treatment of cows that are diagnosed non-pregnant. For example, the exercise by Eddy (1983) described in Chapter 9 combined early diagnosis of non-pregnancy using the milk progesterone test and the use

Table 11.1 A summary of available methods of pregnancy diagnosis.

Test	Stage	Accuracy	Advantages	Disadvantages	Comments
Non-return to service	3 weeks	About 50%	Early	Relies on good oestrus detection	Insemination at 'false oestrus' can lead to abortion
Milk progesterone	3 weeks	Positives 85% Negatives 100%	Early Non-invasive	False positives and later losses	Good test for non-pregnancy
bPAG/PSPB	4 weeks +	Fairly good	Relatively early	Usually needs blood May persist after loss	Can be useful, e.g. in heifers that are hard to palpate
Ultrasound scan	4 weeks +	Up to 100%	Accurate Relatively early	Cost of equipment	Can also detect problems. Recommended
Palpation	6 weeks(?) +	Up to 100%	High accuracy	Possible damage to cow or conceptus	Depends on operator. Early diagnoses especially risky
Oestrone sulphate	15 weeks +	Almost 100%	High accuracy Non-invasive	Only possible after 16–17 weeks	Useful confirmatory test
Mammary development	4 months (heifers)	Up to 100%	Non-invasive	Less useful in lactating cows	
Ballottement	30 weeks +	Positives 100%	Cost	Late	Little practical value in on-farm fertility management

of prostaglandin very effectively, as did the SAC procedure using scanning in heifers described above.

The general cost benefit of the use of pregnancy diagnosis is very difficult to assess since many influencing factors vary from farm to farm. However, if regular pregnancy diagnosis is combined with efficient oestrus detection, a high standard of management and prompt action on non-pregnant cows, then it is likely to be extremely cost effective.

References

Arthur, G.H., Noakes, D.E. & Pearson, H. (1982) *Reproduction and Veterinary Obstetrics*, 5th edn. Baillière Tindall, London.

Boyd, J.S. (1991) *In Practice*, **13**, 109.

Eddy, R.G. (1983) *British Veterinary Journal*, **139**, 104.

Groves, D.J., Sauer, M.J., Rayment, P., Foulkes, J.A. & Morris, B.A. (1990) *Journal of Endocrinology*, **126**, 217–222.

Humblot, P. (2001) *Theriogenology*, **56**, 1417–1433.

Marshall, J.F., Barrett, D.C., Logue, D.N., Ball, P.J.H. & Mihm, M. (2003) *Cattle Practice*, **11**, 151–152.

Morton, H., Morton, D.J. & Ellendorf, F. (1983) *Journal of Reproduction and Fertility*, **68**, 437.

Noakes, D. (1991) In *Bovine Practice* (ed. E. Boden.) Baillière Tindall, London, pp. 65–78.

Patel, O.V., Sulon, J., Beckers, J.F., Takahashi, T., Hirako, M., SaSaki, N.R. & Domeki, I. (1997) *European Journal of Endocrinology*, **137**, 423–428.

Szenci, O., Beckers, J.F., Humblot, P., Sulon, J., Sasser, G., Taverne, M.A., Varga, J., Baltusen, R. & Schekk, G. (1998a) *Theriogenology*, **50**, 77–88.

Szenci, O., Taverne, M.A., Beckers, J.F., Sulon, J., Varga, J., Börzsönyi, L., Hanzen, C. & Schekk, G. (1998b) *Veterinary Record*, **142**, 304–306.

Vaillancourt, D., Bierschwal, C.J., Ogwu, D., Elmore, R.G., Martin, C.E., Sharp, A.J. & Youngquist, R.S. (1981) *Journal of the American Veterinary Medicine Association*, **175**, 466.

Yoshioka, K., Iwamura, S. & Kamomae, H. (1995) *Journal of Veterinary Medical Science*, **57**, 721–725.

Chapter 12
Reproductive Problems

Up to the present chapter we have concentrated largely on a description of reproductive function in 'normal' cattle. However, a number of problems can arise with the reproductive process so that normal function is lost. This can lead to a reduced level of reproductive efficiency or sub-fertility and, in some cases, to total failure of reproduction, or infertility. The most common reproductive problems of the bull and cow are discussed below, although some have been included in previous chapters where appropriate.

Reproductive problems in the bull

With the exception of bulls used for artificial insemination, bovine male fertility receives scant attention. However, the fertilizing ability of the bull is clearly critical in determining the reproductive performance of a herd, irrespective of the fertility status of the cows. Sub-fertility and infertility occur in bulls due to a variety of causes and the most common of these are discussed briefly below.

Congenital problems

The testicles

Testicular hypoplasia or defective testicular development can occur in all breeds and in an American survey was reported to occur in 1.3% of bulls (Carroll *et al.*, 1963). Certain breeds seem to be more prone to the condition, which was very common in Swedish Highland bulls, occurring in up to 25% of animals. The testicles are noticeably smaller than normal, although this may be difficult to define with certainty due to a wide variation between 'normal' animals. The condition may be unilateral or bilateral and in the latter case the bull is likely to be infertile. In any event such bulls should not be used for breeding, because the condition may be of an hereditary nature.

Cryptorchidism is the failure of one or both testicles to descend into the scrotal sac during fetal development. Although testosterone production is not affected, spermatogenesis is inhibited in affected testicles because they are maintained at body temperature. The condition is relatively rare in cattle (approximately 0.1% of bulls) but can be quite common in other species, e.g. the horse.

An additional defect that occasionally occurs (approximately 0.2% of bulls) is the lack of development of segments of the male reproductive tract. An example of this is segmental aplasia or hypoplasia of the Wolffian duct from which the sperm transport system (which transports spermatozoa from the testicles to the urethra) develops (see Chapter 2). This condition is analogous to white heifer disease, discussed later in this chapter. Degeneration of the testicles may occasionally occur but is usually secondary to another disease process or possibly ageing. In this condition the testicles shrink in size and there is a loss of fertilizing ability.

Abnormalities of spermatozoa

The assessment of normal semen characteristics is described in Chapter 10. A variety of morphological abnormalities of sperm occur in the bull and may be associated with infertility. These include detached sperm heads, acrosomal defects, coiled tails and immature sperm each containing a 'proximal droplet' at the junction between the head and midpiece of the sperm. These defects have been described in detail elsewhere (Arthur *et al.*, 1996) and are considered briefly in Chapter 3. Poor quality semen is a major reason for bulls being declared unsuitable for AI purposes. Beef breeds appear to pose a particular problem in this respect.

The penis and prepuce

Prolapse of the prepuce is an eversion of the mucous membrane lining of the prepuce or sheath. It occurs occasionally and appears to be due to congenital hypoplasia of the retractor muscles of the sheath, a feature most common in polled bulls. If this problem is persistent it can lead to chronic infection of the prepuce.

Deviation of the penis occurs in the bull and may be manifested in a variety of ways. For example, lateral, ventral and spiral deviations have all been reported (see Arthur *et al.*, 1996). The causes vary but may often be congenital. For example, persistent attachment of the ventral surface of the penis to the inside of the sheath, a condition known as persistent frenulum, results in ventral deflection of the penis at erection or, in more serious cases, an inability to extrude the penis. Under normal conditions separation of the frenulum is complete by about nine months of age. Although these cases can be treated surgically, such bulls should not be used for pedigree breeding due to the possible hereditary nature of the condition.

Benign virus-induced tumours of the penis and prepuce are common. These may grow quite large and cause irritation and bleed occasionally. The usual outcome is for the tumours to regress spontaneously, although surgical removal may become necessary.

A relatively common traumatic injury is the rupture of the corpus cavernosum penis. The tough membrane surrounding the penile tissue ruptures, usually during service. The resultant haematoma or blood clot normally forms close to the sigmoid flexure. Following this, fibrous adhesions often develop between the penis and prepuce, making extrusion of the penis painful and difficult.

Infections

Infection of the reproductive tract can result in orchitis (inflammation of the testis), epididymitis or seminal vesiculitis. Organisms that have commonly been associated with these conditions are *Brucella abortus* and *Corynebacterium pyogenes*. The symptoms include pain in the inguinal area and elevated body temperature.

Campylobacter (vibrio) fetus and *Trichomonas fetus* colonize the interior of the prepuce and hence infected bulls can transmit these organisms during natural service. However, these infections are rarely associated with lesions of the reproductive tract of the bull. Bovine herpes virus 1 is most commonly associated with infectious bovine rhinotracheitis (IBR) in young cattle but can also cause infection of the penis and prepuce (balanoposthitis) in adult bulls.

Infection of the genital tract with mycoplasmosis is associated with low sperm motility in young bulls. Panangala *et al.* (1981) found that *Mycoplasma bovigenitalium* mixed with bull semen adhered to the spermatozoa and depressed their motility.

Reproductive problems in the cow

As was discussed earlier, reproductive performance in European and North American dairy herds is declining steadily and is more than ever a highly important limiting factor in efficient herd performance. Problems in the female can affect the manifestation and detection of oestrus, the production, transport and fertilization of ova and the transport, implantation and survival of the conceptus.

The underlying causes for these failures can be loosely divided into the categories of developmental, infectious and functional (including injury) problems. However, these distinctions are sometimes poorly demarcated, and tend to overlap. For example, retained placenta, a functional disorder, or injury caused by a difficult calving can predispose the reproductive tract to infection, and this can in turn lead to mechanical damage. The following is a brief summary of the more common clinical problems that result in reproductive failure. Detailed accounts of the causes, diagnosis and treatment of all reproductive problems in cows are covered in more specialized texts.

Developmental problems

Most developmental problems in cattle, as in other species, result from genetic abnormalities, which can either be inherited from one or both parents or result from chromosome damage during oocyte development, fertilization and early embryo development. It is likely that a very high percentage of inherited abnormalities result in fertilization failure or death within a short time of conception, as will be discussed in the relevant sections below. Occasionally, however, calves are born with inherited defects that may affect their survival or reproductive ability. Bovine leukocyte adhesion deficiency (BLAD) is an example of an inherited condition that normally results in the early death of homozygous carriers. It is now thought that even heterozygous carriers tend to have lower milk yields (Jánosa *et al.*, 1999) and the possibility that reproductive performance may also be impaired may warrant investigation. For a review of BLAD see Gerardi (1996). A classic example of an inherited condition that affects reproduction is segmental aplasia of the Müllerian ducts, or white heifer disease. The name derives from the fact that the gene responsible for the condition is associated with white coat colour. The anomaly interferes with the normal development of the Müllerian ducts so that the reproductive tract becomes obstructed. The degree to which the various components of the reproductive tract are affected varies and depends on the time at which development was inhibited. The cow's ovaries are functional and therefore oestrus and ovulation may occur normally. Depending on the site of the obstruction, fertilization, conception and parturition may or may not be possible, since one uterine horn only may be affected. The condition was originally associated with the Shorthorn breed, but is still a recognized problem in currently used breeds, especially the Belgian Blue (Charlier *et al.*, 1996).

As was described in Chapter 2, the oviducts, uterus, cervix and anterior vagina develop from the embryonic Müllerian ducts. Normally, the ducts fuse to form a single cervix and vagina, but occasionally a double cervix is formed (see Fig. 12.1).

Another developmental problem, freemartinism, occurs when a male and a female conceptus are present in the same uterus. It is a well-known phenomenon in cattle, in which there is a tendency for the placentae of twin fetuses to merge, but it is known to occur in other species, and is an increasing problem in sheep (Parkinson *et al.*, 2001). If the placentae merge, the circulatory systems of the twins become interconnected. If one of the twins is a female, the development of the female sexual organs will be affected. This may be due in part to the effect of androgens or other hormones from the male circulation. Rota *et al.* (2002) measured plasma concentrations of anti-Müllerian hormone (AMH) in bovine freemartins. Levels of AMH at birth were very high in males and in freemartins. They remained high in males for the first five months of life, but in the freemartins they rapidly decreased to normal female levels, showing that AMH came from the male twin. The freemartin female is likely to suffer from chimerism, a combination of cells of the two fetuses, and this could in itself be affecting the development of the female tract. Ennis *et al.* (1999) used Y-specific polymerase chain reaction (PCR) primer pairs to detect male cells in the blood of heifers born co-twins to bulls.

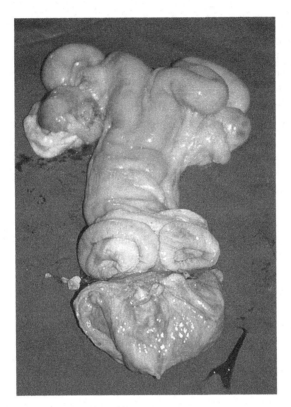

Fig. 12.1 Reproductive tract from a heifer with a double cervix. Both were patent, leading into the uterus. In another heifer, the two fused to form a single passage into the uterus.

Between 1 and 2% of cattle births are twin births. Approximately half of these are heterosexual, i.e. 0.5–1.0%. Approximately 92% of heifers born as heterosexual twins exhibit the freemartin syndrome.

The external genitalia of the freemartin usually appear normal, so that the condition may go unnoticed until it is time to breed the heifer involved. Heifers are affected to varying degrees: the more severe the condition, the more akin to their male counterparts will be the female gonads and reproductive tract. Unlike cows with white heifer disease, those with freemartinism are not likely to have functioning ovaries. It is probable that the condition would be more severe if placental fusion occurred relatively early in development. A typical freemartin reproductive tract is shown in Fig. 12.2 and should be compared with the normal tract shown in Fig. 2.9.

There is no cure for freemartinism, and it is important that the condition is diagnosed at an early age, so that no effort is wasted in rearing a non-productive heifer. When female calves are purchased at a market, a potential buyer may use the 'pencil test', inserting a pen or pencil into the vagina to

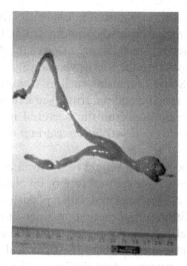

Fig. 12.2 Reproductive tract of a freemartin heifer. Note the underdeveloped uterus and very small ovaries.

determine its length. This may not detect small anatomical abnormalities that could still render the cow infertile. The test of Ennis *et al.* (1999) for the presence of male cells could be useful in practice. Satoh *et al.* (1997) gave pregnant mare serum gonadotrophin and human chorionic gonadotrophin to 4-month dairy heifers. Concentrations of oestradiol-17β and progesterone rose in normal heifers, but there was no response in freemartins. Again, we feel that this test may not detect less severely affected animals, which could nevertheless be infertile or subfertile.

Infectious infertility

Disturbances in reproductive function may occur as the result of non-specific systemic infections. For example, behavioural oestrus may be inhibited in a cow that has a mild systemic disease or embryo loss may be induced by pyrexia resulting from a systemic infection. However, infection of the reproductive tract, particularly the uterus, by non-specific organisms is also very common together with a number of specific pathogens, which selectively affect the reproductive system. The most important examples of these are discussed below.

Endometritis

As was seen in Chapter 7, cattle are unusual in that bacterial contamination occurs in virtually every uterus after parturition. This bacterial load usually decreases during the first three weeks after parturition, but it can last for up to 14 weeks in some cows. In 10–15% of cases, the infection can persist beyond three weeks and worsen, to cause endometritis (Sheldon *et al.*, 2002). Endometritis is an inflammation of the endometrium, the mucous membrane internal lining of the uterus, which occurs as a result of infection by bacteria. Infection normally ascends into the uterus via the vagina particularly at service or around parturition. Some organisms such as *Campylobacter fetus* and *Trichomonas fetus* cause a specific endometritis (see below), but this condition is also caused by non-specific opportunistic bacterial invaders, e.g. *Corynebacterium pyogenes*, *Escherichia coli* and *Fusobacterium necrophorum* (see review by de Bois, 1982).

Endometritis often occurs as a sequel to dystocia and/or retained placenta and may be connected with a decreased rate of involution of the uterus in the postpartum period. It is often associated with a persistent corpus luteum, which tends to make the condition self-perpetuating, since there is no oestrus to help clean out the uterus. LeBlanc *et al.* (2002a) identified clinical endometritis by the presence of purulent uterine discharge or cervical diameter >7.5 cm after 20 days in milk, or by a mucopurulent discharge after 26 days in milk. Many cases were not identified unless vaginoscopy was used. Cows with clinical endometritis between 20 and 33 days after calving took 27% longer to become pregnant, and were 1.7 times more likely to be culled for reproductive failure than cows without endometritis. Reist *et al.* (2003) found that raised milk acetone concentrations (>0.40 mmol/litre) were associated with a 3.2 times higher risk of endometritis. This suggests that metabolic disorder may predispose to, or be associated with, the uterine infection, and also provides a possible means of identifying cows at risk so that appropriate interventions can be considered.

Potential treatments can be divided into (1) systemic antibiotic treatment, (2) uterine infusion, (3) administration of oestrogen to induce uterine response to the infection and (4) injection of prostaglandin to induce oestrus, so that the uterus is cleansed naturally.

Systemic treatments tend to be less favoured, except as an adjunct to other treatments. Oestrogen dominance is known to enhance uterine resistance to infection, but there is little objective evidence that oestrogen therapy alone is effective, although some clinicians favour it. Uterine infusion and/or prostaglandin injection are therefore treatments of choice. Iodine-based infusions have fallen from favour because they may cause irritation and necrosis. Heuwieser *et al.* (2000) compared (1) an intrauterine infusion of 100 ml of a 2% polycondensated m-cresolsulphuric acid formaldehyde solution, (2) an intrauterine infusion of 125 ml of a 20% eucalyptus compositum solution and (3) injection with an analogue of $PGF_{2\alpha}$. Prostaglandin treatment was more effective than the other treatments in terms of oestrus detection efficiency, interval to first service and days open. Not surprisingly, LeBlanc *et al.* (2002b) reported that in endometritic cows with no palpable corpus luteum, prostaglandin treatment was ineffective and, indeed, was associated with a significant reduction in pregnancy rate. They also suggested that, based on criteria associated with subsequent pregnancy rate, treatment of postpartum endometritis should be reserved for cases diagnosed after 26 days postpartum.

Prevention of endometritis is dependent on routine hygiene particularly at the time of calving. It is important that cows are kept clean and that calving boxes are cleaned and disinfected and liberally bedded with clean straw.

Pyometra

This condition is due to an accumulation of pus inside the uterus and usually occurs in association with persistence of the corpus luteum. Pyometra can occur as a sequel to chronic endometritis, and bovine herpesvirus-4 has been identified as one of the causative micro-organisms (Frazier *et al.*, 2002). It may also result from the death of an embryo or fetus with subsequent infection by *C. pyogenes*. The uterus is under the influence of progesterone from the corpus luteum and the cervix is distended. Release of $PGF_{2\alpha}$ is prevented due to endometrial damage. The uterine horns are invariably distended, although to a variable degree. However, the condition is seldom accompanied by systemic illness. The situation may persist undetected for a considerable time since the animal may be thought to be pregnant. Oestrogens followed by oxytocin have been used to treat the condition, but $PGF_{2\alpha}$ is probably more effective.

Specific infective organisms of the female reproductive tract

Campylobacter fetus

This bacterium was formerly known as *Vibrio fetus*. The disease it causes is known as campylobacteriosis or vibriosis. As its name implies, the organism can cause abortion of the fetus. It has been implicated as a cause of embryo or early fetal loss between 25 and 60 days after natural service, in a herd being monitored by means of milk progesterone profiles. In a smaller proportion of cows, abortion may occur at around five months. In the non-pregnant cow the disease can cause endometritis. The organism can be transmitted between cows by means of the bull that serves them. Infected cows eventually become immune to the disease and will resume normal fertility. The organism is sensitive to antibiotics, so that infected bulls can be treated successfully. The use of AI and its attendant precautions has considerably reduced the incidence of the disease in developed countries in the last few decades.

Trichomonas fetus

This protozoan organism is a specific pathogen of the bovine prepuce, vagina and uterus. Infection in the female is characterized by irregular oestrous cycles, low conception rates, vulval discharge, early abortion and pyometra. The incidence of the disease in many countries has been reduced by the widespread use of AI.

Neospora

Neospora caninum infection of the reproductive tract can cause fetal death and later abortions in dairy herds (Crawshaw & Brocklehurst, 2003) and in beef herds (Waldner *et al.*, 1999). Boger & Hattel (2003) considered that fetal neosporosis might be involved in many undiagnosed cases of bovine abortion. Maley *et al.* (2003) concluded that the placenta plays a central role in the pathogenesis and epidemiology of the infection. The parasite may attack the fetus directly, but the maternal and fetal inflammatory responses may also be damaging.

Mycoplasmas

Various mycoplasmas are known to infect the reproductive tract and may cause various reproductive problems. Specifically, *Ureaplasma diversum* lives on urea and is to be found in the vagina, particularly posterior to the urethral opening, where it can cause lesions. It has been shown to cause reproductive disease in cattle, including beef replacement heifers (e.g. Sanderson *et al.*, 2000). For a brief review of the classification, habitat and characteristics of *Ureaplasma*, and the pathogenesis, transmission, clinical syndromes, diagnosis, immunity and treatment of *Ureaplasma diversum* infections in cattle see Miller *et al.* (1994).

Since these organisms could be carried from the posterior vagina into the uterus at artificial insemination, it is recommended that a disposable plastic sheath ('chamise sanitaire') is always used to protect the insemination pipette until it is inserted into the cervix.

Brucellosis

This disease occurs due to infection by the bacterium *Brucella abortus*. Until recently it was probably the most common cause of abortion in cattle in the UK. It is also the cause of undulant fever in man.

Cattle usually become infected by the ingestion of contaminated material, e.g. vaginal discharges, dead fetuses and placentae. The predilection sites for the organisms are the cotyledons in the female and the testes in the male. Transmission of *Brucella* organisms via semen is of doubtful significance, except where fresh semen is inseminated directly into the uterus. Abortion usually occurs between seven and eight months of gestation. This is often followed by placental retention and endometritis. Most cows will remain chronically infected but usually abort only once.

Diagnosis is based on isolation of the organism in the fetus and placenta and the detection of antibodies in serum, milk or semen. Serological diagnosis of the disease was for some years confounded in the UK by the use of the strain-19 *Brucella* vaccine in heifer calves between three and six months of age. New vaccines have since been developed that cause negligible interference with diagnostic serology (Schurig *et al.*, 2002).

The first phase of the eradication of bovine brucellosis began in the UK with the Brucellosis (Accredited Herds) Scheme in 1967 using slaughter of serological reactors as the major means of control. In 1970 it was estimated that 0.4% of all bovine parturitions in the UK (approximately 18000 abortions per year) were abortions due to *Brucella abortus*. However, by 1981 the whole country was attested with almost all herds free of infection and the UK is now considered to be free of the infection. Similar progress has been made in other western countries. In the USA, efforts to eradicate brucellosis caused by *Brucella abortus* began in 1934. As of 31 December 2000, for the first time in the history of the brucellosis programme, there were no affected cattle herds in the USA. However, brucellosis has a variable, sometimes quite lengthy incubation period, so it is expected that additional affected herds will be disclosed (Ragan, 2002).

Other infections affecting reproduction

Many systemic infections of female cattle can affect reproduction in a variety of ways. For example, the resultant illness can cause stress, which can affect various aspects of reproduction, or a raised temperature, which may damage the embryo (see below). The following are only selected examples of such infections.

Infectious bovine rhinotracheitis (IBR) is caused by bovine herpesvirus-1 (BHV-1) in cattle and is similar to cattle flu, caused by the influenza A virus. A further viral infection, bovine virus diarrhoea (BVD), is characterized by diarrhoea, as the name suggests, and also by the birth of persistently infected calves. All three infections are thought to affect reproduction, possibly because of the associated fever and consequent damage to the young embryo. Biuk-Rudan *et al.* (1999), for example, have demonstrated the prevalence of antibodies to IBR and BVD viruses in dairy cows with reproductive disorders, and we have monitored particularly high incidences of detectable embryo and fetal loss in dairy cows with evidence of IBR infection in two herds and BVD infection in one herd. Cows in their first lactation had an abnormally high incidence of loss (Ball, 1997). It is suggested that, since they were reared separately from the main herd, they may not have developed resistance to endemic viral infections, and therefore are particularly susceptible to them. This indicates that, apart from any other precautions, young stock should not be overprotected from infections in the milking herd.

Vaccination is available, and advisable, against IBR (Makoschey & Keil, 2000; van Drunen Littel-van den Hurk *et al.*, 2001) and BVD. The latter virus is more problematic, since vaccination against one strain may not give protection against another. Some BVD type 1 vaccines offer some cross protection against BVD type 2, but specific BVD type 2 vaccines are beginning to become available.

Bacterial infections that cause general ill health in various species and which can specifically affect reproduction in cattle include leptospirosis – mainly

L. hardjobovis, prajitno and *pomona*. Their effects include embryo and early fetal death. *Leptospira* infections can be treated with antibiotics (Alt *et al.*, 2001) and a number of vaccines are available.

Mycotic infections

Fungal infections, particularly those caused by *Aspergillus fumigatus* on mouldy feeds such as poorly made hay and silage, are generally thought to cause abortions fairly late in pregnancy. However, there is some evidence that aflatoxins originating from such moulds can also cause fetal losses at a much earlier stage.

Functional subfertility

Impairment or failure of reproduction can affect any of the following:

- production and ovulation of viable ova
- ovum transport
- expression and detection of oestrus
- fertilization
- the fertilized ovum and early embryo stage (0–25 days after fertilization)
- the late embryo/early fetus stage (26–60 days)
- the late fetus stage (especially abortion in the third trimester of pregnancy).

All of these functions are susceptible to a variety of factors, of which the most important can be grouped under (1) nutrition, (2) other forms of stress, and (3) infection, which has been dealt with separately.

Nutrition

The importance of nutrition to good reproductive performance will have become apparent in discussion of the ovarian cycle in Chapter 4. The specific effects of various dietary constituents on reproductive performance are still poorly understood, in spite of years of research. There are many conflicting reports on the effects that deficiencies of β-carotene and selenium, to name but two, have on reproductive performance. Their effects interact with so many dietary and other factors, that it is extremely difficult to assess the effect of any one of many dietary components in isolation. In any case, detailed discussion of all aspects of nutritional influences on reproduction is beyond the scope of this book. For more comprehensive coverage, see McClure (1994) and BSAS (1995).

However, it is quite clear that poor metabolic status, and negative energy balance in particular, can compromise a number of aspects of reproductive performance. This is related to the natural metabolic mechanisms that tend to direct nutrients towards milk production at the expense of other functions such as reproduction. During periods of negative energy balance, which can last up to 20 weeks after calving in very high yielding cows, body tissue is mobilized to make up the shortfall, releasing non-esterified fatty acids (NEFAs) and ketone bodies into the circulation. If cows are over-fat at calving, there is increased mobilization, leading to appetite depression, which in turn increases the magnitude of the negative energy balance. High crude protein levels, typical of present-day cow diets, can lead to an excess of rumen degradable protein in relation to available fermentable metabolizable energy. This leads to an increase in the production of ammonia, which requires energy for its detoxification. This will also worsen the negative energy balance as will high concentrate to forage ratios in the diet, which can lead to acidosis and thus to reduced dry matter intake.

The effect of negative energy balance is mediated mainly through a deficiency in IGF-I and insulin levels, which are in turn associated with low concentrations of plasma leptin. Block *et al.* (2001) reported that postpartum negative energy balance and the associated low leptin levels could be counteracted by not milking the cows under study and they concluded that the energy deficit of postpartum cows causes a sustained reduction in plasma leptin, designed to benefit early lactating dairy cows by promoting a faster increase in feed intake and by diverting energy from non-vital functions such as reproduction. The resultant low in IGF-I and insulin levels affects, respectively, follicle proliferation and oestrogen production (Wathes *et al.*, 2003). Poor oestradiol secretion compromises LH release, affecting ovulation and subsequent luteal development (Starbuck *et al.*, 2000).

Stress

Stress can be defined as the inability of an animal to cope with its environment, so that it fails to achieve its genetic potential in one or more areas, including growth rate, milk yield, disease resistance and fertility (Dobson & Smith, 2000). Various stressful factors can adversely affect fertility. Lameness (e.g., Collick *et al.*, 1989), mastitis (e.g., Huszenicza *et al.*, 1998) and milk fever (e.g., Borsberry & Dobson, 1989) have all been shown to have significant adverse effects on reproductive parameters such as calving to first service and calving to conception intervals.

Even the stress of a change in social status within a dairy herd has been shown to affect reproductive performance (Dobson & Smith 2000; see Table 12.1), although the effect is confounded with the increased lameness associated with lowered social status. Using ewes as a model, Smith *et al.* (1997) transported a group of animals for two hours and measured an immediate constant increase in arginine vasopressin (AVP) and corticotrophin-releasing hormone (CRH) secretion. Both transport in ewes and ACTH administration in heifers (Dobson *et al.*, 2000) reduced LH pulse frequency and magnitude, which could in turn affect oestrogen production by the developing follicle. As with negative

Table 12.1   The effect of social status. (From Dobson and Smith, 2000.)

	Change in social status	
	Increase	*Decrease*
Calving to conception (days)	97	143
Inseminations per conception	1.6	2.2
Milk yield (kg/day)	+0.58	–1.03
Somatic cell count ('000/ml)	–18	+371
Difference in lameness score	–0.021	+0.54

energy balance, this could have repercussions for ovulation and subsequent corpus luteum function. The effects may be mediated, at least in part, at pituitary level because exogenous ACTH, or transport, reduces the amount of LH released by challenges with exogenous GnRH.

Specific reproductive problems

Dystocia

Dystocia may be defined as difficulty or prolongation of parturition as opposed to normal parturition described in Chapter 6. Causes of dystocia can be classified broadly as maternal or fetal in origin and these are summarized in Fig. 12.3.

Maternal causes may be due to anatomical or pathological defects in the birth canal, which includes the bony pelvis, uterus, cervix, vagina or vulva (see Fig. 12.3). Failure of uterine contractions (inertia) is the most likely defect of the expulsive forces and may be considered as being primary or secondary. Secondary inertia usually occurs as a result of fatigue following a prolonged second-stage labour. Primary uterine inertia can arise due to intrinsic defects in the myometrium, e.g. toxic degeneration and senility or abnormalities in hormone release. A common cause of primary uterine inertia and dystocia is the lack of calcium ions that occurs in the onset of parturient hypocalcaemia (milk fever). Overcondition of the cow at calving predisposes her to dystocia and it is important to try to aim for calving in moderate condition (around 3 on a scale of 0–5) to avoid calving problems and the damage they may cause.

However, in the cow the most common causes of dystocia are fetal in origin and these are invariably due to either fetal oversize or abnormal disposition of the fetus. As discussed in Chapter 6, at calving the fetus is normally dispositioned so that the forelegs appear first followed by the head and then the rest of the body and finally the hind limbs (see Fig. 6.2). This is known as anterior (forward) presentation in the dorsal (upright) position and in an extended posture. Hence presentation refers to the direction in which the long axis of the calf is orientated, while position denotes whether the calf is upright, on its side (lateral) or upside down (ventral). Posture, on the other hand, denotes the

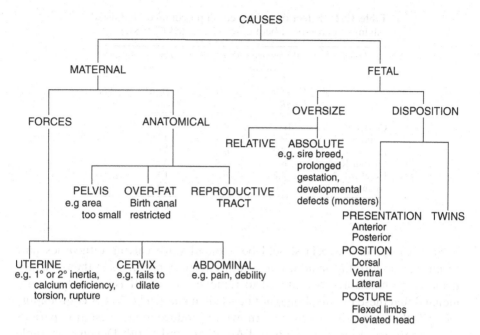

Fig. 12.3 Common causes of dystocia in cows.

configuration of the limbs and head (flexed or extended). The most common abnormalities of presentation in the cow are posterior or breech presentation (posterior with the hind legs forward), whilst the most common postural abnormalities are flexion of the forelimbs and lateral deviation of the head. If any of these abnormalities of fetal disposition are suspected then veterinary help should be sought immediately. The presence of twin fetuses may also be complicated by dispositional abnormalities.

Perhaps the most important cause of dystocia from a cattle breeding point of view is that of fetal oversize, which may be considered to be either 'relative' or 'absolute' (Fig. 12.3). The term 'relative' refers to the size of the fetus in relation to the size of the dam. For example, the dam may be a small heifer, but if the calf is of normal size for that breed it may be too large to pass through the maternal birth canal.

Absolute fetal oversize may occur as a result of gross developmental abnormalities, i.e. the development of monsters. A discussion of such abnormalities is outside the scope of this book, but these include the occurrence of hydrocephalus, anasarca and schistosomes. Alternatively, absolute fetal oversize may occur simply because the calf is large. A major factor influencing the size or weight of the fetus is the breed of sire. Problems often arise with the use of beef bulls. The effect of sire breed on calving difficulties as reported by an MLC survey is given in Table 12.2 and shows that Charolais and Simmental bulls produce the highest percentage of difficult calvings in crossbred beef cows.

Table 12.2   Effect of sire breed on percentage of assisted calvings in crossbred beef cows. (From MLC, 1981.)

Sire breed	Percentage assisted calvings		Percentage calf mortality	
	Hereford × *Friesian*	*Blue-* *Grey*	*Hereford ×* *Friesian*	*Blue-* *Grey*
Charolais	10.1	9.0	5.1	4.4
Simmental	9.7	8.9	4.7	3.7
Limousin	7.9	6.4	4.9	3.9
Lincoln Red	6	4.8	3.5	2.4
Hereford	4.2	3.3	1.8	1.3
Angus	2.0	1.1	1.5	1.1

Such causes of dystocia should be avoided since calving difficulties may result in calf mortality, in addition to future fertility problems in the dam, particularly if much force is required to remove the calf. It is certainly recommended that these breeds should not be used on maiden heifers. A confounding factor is that some sire breeds are known to produce longer gestation periods than others, e.g. Limousin, Blonde d'Aquitaine and South Devon (see Table 5.2). Therefore this factor tends to predispose to heavier calf weights.

The breed of dam is also important in determining the incidence of dystocia. The Friesian cow, for example, has been shown to have poorer calving ability than other dairy breeds (Stables, 1980). An MLC survey of the percentage assisted calvings in Hereford × Friesian cows compared to Blue-Grey cows showed that the latter had superior calving characteristics (see Table 12.2). Most calves born to purebred Belgian Blue cattle have to be delivered by Caesarean section.

Fetal oversize (relative or absolute) occurs as a consequence of the relationship between the size of the fetus and that of the maternal pelvis. A number of studies have been carried out where the area of the maternal pelvis has been measured in relation to the incidence of dystocia. However, it is difficult to apply such predictive techniques to reduce the level of dystocia in practice without some additional control over the selection of sires used and hence of calf size. The problem of fetal oversize has also been encountered following in vitro fertilization (see Thompson & Peterson, 2000).

One of the most serious consequences of dystocia is the death of the calf. Not surprisingly, Peeler *et al.* (1994) found that calf mortality and dystocia were strongly associated. Also physical damage to the dam resulting from dystocia can have a serious effect on future reproductive performance and it can lead to other problems such as endometritis (Kruip *et al.*, 2001), vulval discharge and mastitis (Peeler *et al.*, 1994).

The management of dystocia problems will not be considered here, apart from a mention of preventative management by avoiding overcondition at calving. It suffices to state that only experienced stockpersons should attempt to interfere in cases of dystocia. If there is any doubt, then veterinary attention should be sought urgently.

Retention of the placenta

Expulsion of the fetal membranes is the third stage of labour and is usually accomplished within 6 hours of parturition. However, in some cows the fetal membranes are not expelled normally but may remain attached to the uterine caruncles for a variable period after parturition. The direct cause of this condition is uncertain, but it is related to a deficiency of myometrial contractions. Consequently, placental retention is usually accompanied and followed by delayed involution of the uterus (Arthur *et al.*, 1996). Retention often occurs as a result of 'premature' birth, which may arise in a variety of circumstances. For example, it is associated with abortion due to infectious causes, Caesarean section and pharmacological induction of parturition (see Chapter 6). Peeler *et al.* (1994) reported that twinning was found to be a significant predictor for retained fetal membranes. Pharmacological induction of parturition is also very likely to cause placental retention, and is sometimes used deliberately to study the condition and possible treatments (e.g., Königsson *et al.*, 2001). There is evidence that retention is related to an endocrine imbalance and low plasma oestrogen concentrations have been implicated. The incidence of retained placenta following normal unassisted calvings appears to be of the order of 8–11%.

As with dystocia, retained placenta can predispose to impairment of subsequent reproductive performance. The fertility of such cows is often reduced in terms of a delayed calving to first service interval, calving to conception interval and pregnancy rate to first insemination. Peeler *et al.* (1994) found that the problem of retained fetal membranes was an important risk factor for vulval discharge and increased the risk of mastitis, which can in turn lead to stress and impaired reproductive function. Tefera *et al.* (2001) reported that placental retention was followed by significantly increased periods of abnormal vaginal discharge, intervals to uterine involution, intervals to first ovulation and rates of endometritis as compared with cows that were not affected. They also found that bPSPB blood concentrations were higher in cows with placental retention and suggested that this could be a useful diagnostic aid. The aetiology, pathogenesis and economic losses associated with bovine retained placenta are reviewed in Laven & Peters (1996).

The treatment of retained placenta remains a controversial issue amongst veterinarians. Since the condition is associated with a lack of myometrial activity, agents that stimulate contractions appear to be quite effective, particularly if applied within a day or two of calving (Arthur *et al.*, 1996). Therefore oxytocin and $PGF_{2\alpha}$ are often used for this purpose, although Hickey *et al.* (1984) failed to show any advantage of oxytocin treatment. Manual removal of the placenta by detaching it from the cotyledonary attachments, followed by intrauterine antibiotic therapy, is often carried out, usually after day 3 when separation is more easily effected. In the UK, manual removal is still carried out by a large number of veterinarians, but it is unlikely to be as effective as it may appear (see review by Peters & Laven, 1996). The procedure may be considered undesirable due to possible introduction of infection into the uterus and trauma to the endometrium. These authors favoured the use of systemic antibiotics only, to control possible infection. Apparently this should not be administered too soon, since Königsson *et al.* (2001) found that antibiotic treatment of cows before placental shedding postponed detachment of the placenta.

Inactive ovaries

Following parturition the cow undergoes a variable period of acyclicity or sexual quiescence before reproductive cycles recommence. This acyclic period can be said to be abnormally long when ovulation has not occurred by day 50 postpartum. However, this is quite clearly an arbitrary definition. Rather than being an abnormality, a long period could possibly be regarded as a physiological strategy on the part of the cow to delay further conception while adverse environmental conditions prevail. The factors affecting the length of the acyclic period and its endocrinological control were discussed in detail in Chapter 7.

From the discussion in Chapter 7 and above, it is apparent that ovarian acyclicity basically results from the failure of a follicle to ovulate, even though a succession of follicles is continuing to grow and regress. This may be manifested as an abnormally long delay to the first postpartum ovulation (sometimes termed delayed ovulation type 1 or DOV1) or to a failure to re-ovulate some time after cycles have started (DOV2; see Wathes *et al.*, 2003). DOV2 can result in periods of activity from as little as 7–10 days (if an ovulation occurs from among the next wave of follicles) up to many weeks. Postpartum uterine bacterial contamination can have a short-term effect on follicular development and selection, especially in the ovary ipsilateral to the previously pregnant horn (Sheldon *et al.*, 2002), but the major causes of DOV1 and DOV2 appear to be (1) severe negative energy balance, mediated through IGF-I and insulin levels (Wathes *et al.*, 2003), and (2) stress, interfering with LH release patterns (Dobson & Smith, 2000).

The problem is thus best dealt with through management procedures to optimize feeding strategies and to minimize stress in order to create the conditions likely to favour the onset and continuation of ovarian cyclicity. However, hormone treatments have been investigated and found to be efficacious in initiating ovulation and reducing calving to conception intervals (Ball, 1982; see Table 12.3 and Fig. 12.4). Gümen & Seguin (2003), in a study of early postpartum cows with inactive ovaries, reported that nearly all cows (95%) responded to GnRH treatment with a release of LH but only 45% (10/22) responded with an ovulation and subsequent formation of a corpus luteum. As might be expected, there was no response to $PGF_{2\alpha}$ administration.

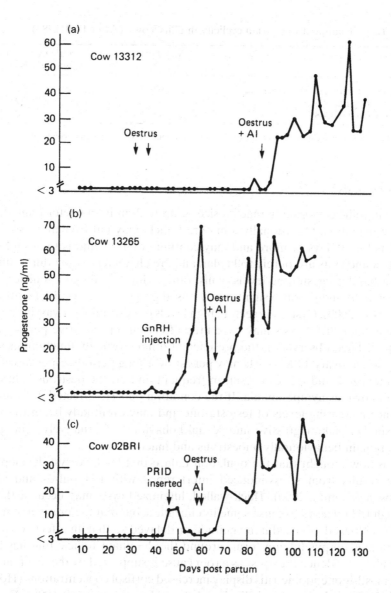

Fig. 12.4 Milk progesterone profiles of three postpartum dairy cows. Cow 13312 (a) resumed ovarian cycles naturally but not until between days 80 and 90 postpartum. Cow 13265 (b) was injected with 500 μg GnRH on day 46 postpartum and underwent a rapid rise in progesterone concentration. Cow 02BRI (c) was fitted with a PRID on day 46 postpartum and showed oestrus after its removal. Both cows in (b) and (c) conceived to AI given at the induced oestrus.

Table 12.3   Treatment of ovarian cyclicity in dairy cows. (After Ball, 1982)

Treatment	No. of cows	Calving to conception interval (days)
No treatment until day 90 postpartum	92	95.3
GnRH (500 µg day 42)	34	88.9
PRID (inserted day 48)	48	81.0[a]

[a] PRID treatment significantly reduced the calving to conception interval compared to control cows.

Ovarian cysts

Ovarian follicles normally reach a size of up to 2 cm in diameter immediately before ovulation. Occasionally a mature follicle may fail to ovulate, so that it persists for 10 days or more and may continue to grow and is then said to be cystic. Some cysts are purely follicular, and are characterized by thin walls and low or basal progesterone levels, whilst others (luteinized cystic follicles) have thicker walls and produce significantly raised progesterone levels (Douthwaite & Dobson, 2000). Cysts may secrete high levels of oestradiol for varying periods of time. Short-lived cysts may have little effect on reproductive performance, and have been observed in the presence of other, normally functioning, structures on the ovary. Other cysts may persist over long periods, especially if they are luteinized, and this can result in frequent and erratic oestrous behaviour, often known as nymphomania. If the condition persists, affected cows tend to produce increasing levels of testosterone and may eventually begin to exhibit virilism, i.e. male aggressive and sexual behaviour. Alternatively some cystic cows remain behaviourally anoestrous and inactive.

It is now thought that the ovulation failure that leads to cyst development often results from stress-induced interference with LH pulses and surges (Dobson & Smith, 2000). Thick-walled, luteinized cysts may occur if there is enough LH released to cause some luteinization, but that the pre-ovulatory LH surge is blocked, reduced in magnitude or delayed so that, in effect, a partially functioning corpus luteum forms around the dominant follicle that has failed to ovulate. Evidence for stress as a root cause is supported by the fact that cows with mastitis or endometritis display increased cortisol concentrations (Hockett *et al.*, 2000) and extended follicular phases (Huszenicza *et al.*, 1998). Furthermore, when ACTH was used to mimic stress effects, pulses and surges of LH were reduced and persistent follicles resulted (Dobson *et al.*, 2000).

Recent reports indicate an incidence of cysts resulting from ovulation failure of between 6 and 19% (Hooijer *et al.*, 2001; Silvia *et al.* 2002), a considerable increase on figures reported in the 1970s. Milk progesterone profile studies at the Scottish Agricultural College (P.J.H. Ball, personal communication) indicated that certain cows had an inherent propensity to luteinized cysts in particular, suggesting that there may be a degree of inheritance. Hooijer *et al.* (2001) calculated sufficient levels of heritability for cysts in general to suggest that the condition could be bred into cows along with selection for milk yield.

Selecting out affected cows has significantly reduced the incidence of cystic ovarian disease in Scandinavia. It is not clear whether selection favours endocrine or anatomical factors specifically causing cysts, or simply a greater susceptibility to stress.

If the cystic ovary condition is partly hereditary this questions the desirability of treatment, since if such animals breed successfully the condition would be more likely to persist in future generations. Both GnRH and human chorionic gonadotrophin (HCG) – an LH-like protein hormone – may be used to treat ovarian cysts, although prostaglandin may be more successful if significant luteinization has already occurred. Progesterone-releasing intravaginal devices have also been used with limited success (e.g. Douthwaite & Dobson 2000). López-Gatius *et al.* (2001) reported that cows with persistent follicles could be successfully synchronized and inseminated at a fixed time using progesterone, GnRH and $PGF_{2\alpha}$ but showed a limited response to treatment with GnRH plus $PGF_{2\alpha}$.

Luteinized cysts tend to re-occur after treatment – another reason for culling rather than curing if there is an option. If the condition is associated with nymphomania, the cow can be used usefully as an aid to detecting oestrus in her herdmates until she is sold.

The incidence of cystic ovaries is considered to be much lower in beef than in dairy cattle.

Prolonged luteal function

In the ovarian cycle the corpus luteum normally begins to regress on day 16 or 17. Occasionally and in the absence of pregnancy the corpus luteum may persist for a longer period. Such cases are often accompanied by uterine problems such as endometritis or pyometra and are explained by a failure of the luteolytic mechanism. Also the persistence of a corpus luteum can accompany the presence of a mummified fetus. Furthermore, prolonged luteal function has been recorded in 1.5% of non-pregnant dairy cows in the absence of any detectable uterine abnormality (Bulman & Lamming, 1977) and in these cases the cause is uncertain.

Ball & McEwan (1998) showed that cows that started to cycle less than 25 days after calving were much more likely to develop prolonged luteal function. This may be due to the fact that the first ovulation, or luteinization of a follicle, occurred before the uterus was sufficiently involuted to control luteolysis (see Table 12.4 and Fig. 12.5).

Cases of prolonged luteal function are sometimes referred to as 'cystic'. This is incorrect since they may not contain a fluid-filled antrum or cavity and, in any case, corpora lutea of normal life span very often have such a cavity (see Fig. 12.6). Prolonged luteal function has also often been diagnosed in cows that have not been observed in oestrus. A more probable explanation is that the corpus luteum is normal but that the cow's oestrous period was missed. Many cases of prolonged luteal function, especially if they accompany endometritis

Table 12.4 Incidence of prolonged luteal function as determined by milk progesterone measurements. (Nineteen other cows that had prolonged delays to start of cycling or that subsequently developed abnormalities such as cystic follicles are not included.) (From Ball and McEwan 1997.)

Days to start of ovarian activity	No. of cows	Prolonged luteal function	
		(No.)	(%)
<25	73	18	25[a]
25–45	34	0	0[b]

[a,b] Proportions differ significantly (χ^2 test $P < 0.01$).

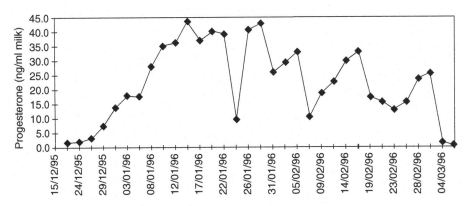

Fig. 12.5 Progesterone profile of cow 488 which calved on 15/12/95 and was injected with prostaglandin, successfully treating prolonged luteal function, on 2/3/96.

or pyometra, can cause seriously long delays to conception, but this is not invariably the case (Taylor *et al.*, 2003).

Possible treatments have been discussed for endometritis and pyometra, which is normally associated with persistent luteal function. Whether or not the condition is associated with uterine infection, the best approach is to remove the corpus luteum, which should bring the cow into oestrus and thus clean out the uterus. In the past it has been common practice to manually enucleate the corpus luteum per rectum in order to advance the onset of oestrus. However, this is not now favoured due to the high risk of haemorrhage and/or the formation of fibrous adhesions. Injection of prostaglandin is a more acceptable method (Fig. 12.5).

Ovaro-bursal adhesions

These occur as a formation of fibrous bands between the surface of the ovary and the ovarian bursa. Their severity varies from the presence of a few small

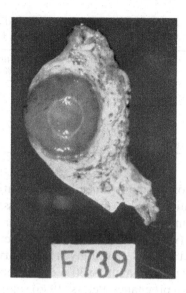

Fig. 12.6 Section through a cow's ovary containing a mature corpus luteum. Note presence of cavity in centre of luteal tissue.

strands of fibrous tissue to severe adhesions where the ovary may be embedded in a mass of fibrous tissue.

The most likely causes of adhesions are excessive follicular haemorrhage at ovulation, trauma to the ovary and bursa during rectal examination and infection ascending from the uterus. The latter is most likely to occur in the postpartum cow suffering from endometritis. Damage during calving, especially in overfat cows, can also cause bleeding and the subsequent formation of adhesions. If the problem is severe then occlusion of the fallopian tubes may result, preventing passage of the ovum after ovulation. In the case of unilateral adhesions the cow may still be fertile, shedding ova normally from the contralateral ovary. The presence of ovaro-bursal adhesions may be difficult to diagnose in the live animal, but their presence might be suspected in cows showing persistent regular returns to oestrus.

Failure of pregnancy

Fertilization failure and early embryonic loss

A number of experiments, some of them based on the recovery of embryos after slaughter at various stages after insemination, have shown that under ideal conditions a very high proportion of ova produced at ovulation become fertilized, but that many embryos are lost during the early days of pregnancy (reviewed by Ayalon, 1984). However, the situation has changed since these experiments were reported and, in any case under farm conditions, the average

Table 12.5 Approximate pregnancy rates and cumulative loss rates in cattle. (Data reviewed by Peters, 1996.)

Day	Pregnancy rate (%)	Cumulative loss (%)
0	90	10
13	81	19
19	66	34
42	60	40
280 (calving rate)	55	45

fertilization rate is almost certainly much lower, and it is impossible to distinguish between fertilization failure and very early loss. Progesterone concentrations are of no help in making this distinction. By day 19 only about 50% of cows are still pregnant (we quoted 60–65% in earlier editions!), and by day 40 the figure falls to about 45–50%. Even given a conservative estimate of 75% fertilization rate, this suggests that up to 30% of all embryos conceived are lost during the first 40 days of pregnancy. Peters (1996) summarized cumulative loss rates extracted from the literature and these are shown in Table 12.5. They give a good idea of the relative importance of losses at various stages, but even these are probably optimistic by current standards.

A number of management factors can affect the success of fertilization, with treatment at and around the time of service and insemination technique being important. Poor timing of insemination can affect the chances of conception. Apparently, spermatozoa from different bulls take different lengths of time to capacitate in the female tract, so that optimal insemination times may be different for different bulls. This may explain why mixtures of sperm from different bulls (see Chapter 10) can be more fertile on average than the semen from any of the individuals used alone.

Even if management and procedures are of the highest order, some fertilization failure and early loss is inevitable, as shown, for example, by embryo recovery experiments. Poor bull fertility only explains a proportion of this failure. One of the risks at fertilization is polyspermy. This results when two or more spermatozoa are able to penetrate the zona pelucida, so that the resulting ovum has an extra complement of male-derived chromosomes. The problem is often encountered during in vitro fertilization procedures (e.g., Mizushima & Fukui, 2001) and can sometimes be traced to the bull used for the insemination (Saacke *et al.*, 2000).

Once fertilization has occurred, the embryo has to make its way to the uterus for subsequent implantation and to develop sufficiently to produce enough interferon tau (IFNτ) to prevent luteolysis at about day 17. Any failure in this process could be due to a defect in the embryo itself and/or a problem with the maternal environment. Whilst it has been claimed that the majority of embryo loss in cows is due to genetic defects (Bishop, 1964), there is clearly a lack of cytogenetic evidence for this. In more recent studies only 3 and 14% of early embryos collected from heifers and cows respectively during the first few days of pregnancy showed genetic abnormalities (Gayerie, 1983; Maurer & Echternkamp, 1985), figures that are much too low to account for the rate of embryo loss that actually occurs.

It is now established that the major problem is a deficient maternal environment, mediated by inadequate luteal function within the first few days of conception. As was seen in Chapter 5, Starbuck *et al.* (2001) showed that cows with 'adequate' milk progesterone levels (>3 ng/ml) on day 5 after mating had pregnancy rates over 50%, compared to less than 10% for cows with <1 ng/ml. Marshall *et al.* (2003) found that milk progesterone levels on day 6 after insemination were almost twice as high in cows subsequently diagnosed pregnant as in those diagnosed non-pregnant.

Three possible approaches in the prevention of these early losses are:

- IFNτ supplementation. This is appropriate around the time of expected luteolysis, and would obviously be ineffective if the embryo had already been lost (see Peters, 1996).
- To attempt to enhance luteal function by injection of HCG (LH-like) or GnRH, both of which may exert some luteotrophic effect. Use of GnRH would appear to be more successful than HCG. Results have been variable, but overall there seem to be positive effects (see Peters *et al.*, 2000).
- Progesterone supplementation. This is also an effective approach in some cases. In an analysis of 17 studies involving progesterone supplementation before day 6, Mann & Lamming (1999) demonstrated a highly significant 10.3% improvement in pregnancy rate. Later supplementation was much less effective.

Although on average there are clear differences in progesterone levels between subsequently pregnant and subsequently non-pregnant cows, individual variation restricts the usefulness of such measurements to decide which cows should be treated. Marshall *et al.* (2003) measured an increase in milk progesterone levels from day 5–6 of 3 ng/ml in subsequently pregnant cows compared to 1 ng/ml in non-pregnant cows. Further information is needed to confirm that this parameter could be of use in predicting vulnerable cows that could benefit from progesterone supplementation.

Other factors affecting fertilization and the survival of the very early embryo include:

- High intakes of quickly degradable nitrogen, as might occur when grazing heavily fertilized spring grass, lead to high nitrite and urea levels, which can affect ovulation, fertilization and/or the early embryo (up to about 20 days) (see Laven *et al.*, 2002).
- Heat stress (e.g., Wolfenson *et al.*, 2000) can affect ovarian activity through the stress mechanisms already described and can also cause direct damage to the embryo.

In any herd of cows, even where pregnancy rates are typically high, a variable proportion of cows will require three or more inseminations in order to establish a successful pregnancy. Such cows often return to oestrus at regular, 21-day intervals and are thus known as repeat breeders. For reasons mentioned above it is impossible in these cases to determine whether fertilization has failed or whether an embryo has been lost. It is perhaps even more difficult to determine possible causes. Indeed there may not be a problem! Given a highly acceptable conception rate of 70%, on average 30 cows in every 100 will need a second insemination, nine of them will need a third and two or three will need a fourth insemination to conceive. Are those two or three cows problem breeders, or are they just unlucky? They could well be candidates for preventative treatments, but if they are repeat breeders in subsequent lactations they may well have an innate problem which could be inherited, and culling should be considered. Båge *et al.* (2003), using in vitro techniques (see Chapter 13), were able to establish physiological differences between normal and repeat breeder heifers.

Late embryo and early fetal death

Incidence and timing of loss

A number of pregnancy failures also occur beyond about 25 days after conception. These losses are sometimes referred to as detectable embryo or fetal losses, in contrast to those occurring earlier which cannot clearly be distinguished from fertilization failures. The presence of a viable fetus at day 16 is sufficient to extend the life of the corpus luteum, so that progesterone assay techniques can be used to improve the accuracy of monitoring the extent and timing of loss. In studies at the National Institute for Research in Dairying, Reading, (Ball, 1980), fetuses were seen to be expelled in confirmation of milk progesterone evidence (Fig. 12.7).

Early attempts to quantify these losses relied on the detection of oestrus following the fetal loss. Thus if an animal was seen in oestrus 42 days after service, it was not possible to determine whether this was a second ovulation after conception failure, or whether the fetus had just been lost. Therefore it is almost inevitable that there would be an overestimate of the incidence of fetal loss from data collected in this way. Progesterone measurement has helped to overcome this overestimation.

At the same time, control and eradication of certain diseases (e.g., campylobacteriosis) as a result of the introduction of AI has enabled a far higher proportion of conceptuses to survive. Therefore estimates of fetal loss rate based on milk progesterone analyses carried out in the late 1970s and early 1980s range between approximately 5 and 12% of cows, as opposed to figures of approximately 25% estimated two to three decades earlier using non-return rates to oestrus. Since then, however, the situation has worsened considerably, in line with the general trend of worsening fertility. Progesterone profile studies

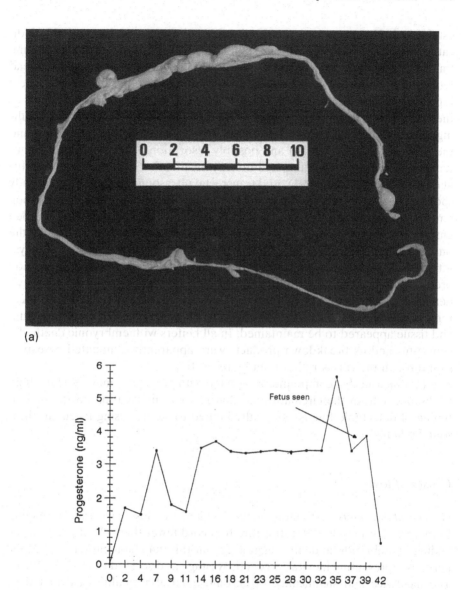

Fig. 12.7 (a) Fetus seen expelled from a milk progesterone monitored cow. (b) Skimmed milk progesterone profile of the cow losing the conceptus shown in (a).

of over 2000 postpartum periods of cows studied in the west of Scotland in the 1990s revealed an incidence of detectable loss of 15–20% (Ball, 1997).

Milk progesterone studies (e.g., Ball, 1980) suggest that almost all of the losses have occurred by day 60 of pregnancy and that they are concentrated around 30–40 days after insemination, at the time that implantation is firmly established. However, progesterone levels may not always be a reliable indicator of the time of loss, because in some cases they may remain high until some time after a loss has occurred. If there was a delay before expulsion of the dead fetus and membranes, or if there was resorption over a period of time, luteal regression would be prevented and the profile would overestimate the age of the conceptus at death. It is possible that there are two types of loss: one resulting in fetal expulsion followed promptly by a rapid drop in progesterone, and the other involving retention and possibly resorption of the dead fetus, maintenance of the corpus luteum, and thus overestimation of the age of the fetus at death. Kastelic *et al.* (1991) used transrectal ultrasound examination to study spontaneous embryonic death, as determined by cessation of heartbeat. When embryonic death was detected prior to day 25, luteal regression preceded embryonic death, whereas when it was detected between days 25 and 40 the onset of luteal regression was detected at least three days (range 3–42 days) after the detection of embryonic death. In heifers in which luteal regression preceded embryonic death the conceptus was lost rapidly, with minimal evidence of degeneration. In heifers in which embryonic death preceded luteal regression there was evidence of conceptus degeneration, but conceptus fluid and tissue appeared to be maintained. In all heifers with embryonic death, the conceptus and its breakdown products were apparently eliminated by expulsion through the cervix rather than by resorption.

Other measurable compounds associated with pregnancy may also take time to disappear from the circulation, so that reliable information on the precise timing of detectable loss is essentially limited to studies using frequent ultrasound scanning.

Causes of loss

Genetic abnormality: estimates of the incidence of loss vary widely, ranging from 4.8 to 26% (Ball, 1997). It is rare to record fewer than 5% of pregnancies ending in embryo/fetal death, suggesting that this may be a basic level of loss, perhaps representing inevitable genetic wastage as discussed by Bishop (1964). The incidence and significance of chromosomal abnormalities as related to embryo/fetal loss are reviewed in Ball (1997), as is the bull's contribution (which in part results from chromosome abnormalities) to such losses.

Some of the cows studied by Ball (1997) were monitored for up to four successive lactations and there was evidence of individual cows being more prone to the problem, suggesting an inherent defect that could be inherited. As with luteinized cystic follicles, it is possible that the condition could have been bred into the cows along with high milk production.

Nutrition: as with early losses, poor nutritional status can cause detectable loss. Cows that lose body condition in early pregnancy are more prone to losses (e.g., Ball & Ecclestone, unpublished). Nutritional effects may be manifested through the level of feeding or through deficiency or imbalance of components of feed, such as energy, minerals, vitamins, etc. The subject is vast and is complicated by interrelationships with other factors, as was highlighted by McClure (1994) in his review of nutritional and metabolic infertility in the cow. The subject will not be pursued further here.

Stress: it may be of interest that we are aware of only one farm in which no embryo losses have been detected in progesterone studies. This was at a monastery in the East Midlands of England, where the cows were extremely well managed and gently treated. At the other end of the scale, Ball (1995) studied the effects of change from pasture to winter housing during a three-week period. He reported that the stress of a fire and atrocious weather conditions caused detectable loss in half of the cows that were between 25 and 60 days pregnant. It is likely that at least some stress-related loss occurs via the pathways that affect progesterone production as discussed above. Stress can be caused by many factors, some of them avoidable, such as changing groups or feeds, housing and treatments such as foot trimming. As far as possible, these should be minimized and avoided during the critical first two months of pregnancy.

Infectious causes: worldwide, infection, whether specific, such as with *Campylobacter fetus venerealis*, or non-specific, is a common cause of fertility problems in cattle, including detectable conceptus loss. The fact that infectious agents can cause the death of the late embryo or early fetus has also been shown by means of experimental infection with, e.g., *Actinomyces pyogenes* and bovine virus diarrhoea (see Ball, 1997).

Pathogens account for some fetal losses even in countries where disease control is well advanced. Campylobacteriosis and infection by bovine herpes 1 virus (IBR) have already been discussed in this context. Another viral disease of increasing importance and associated with fetal loss is that of bovine virus diarrhoea (BVD). In one of the herds in the current Scottish Agricultural College studies, the frequency of loss was greatest in older cows, as would be expected, but there was also a higher proportion of loss in lactations 1 and 2 than in the lactations 3 and 4, as shown in Table 12.6. It is postulated that in

Table 12.6 Incidence of embryo/fetal loss as estimated using milk progesterone profiles.

Lactation	Detectable loss	
	(No.)	*(%)*
1	5	23
2	6	13
3	1	3
4	2	17
5–10	7	28

such cases cows already established in the herd have developed resistance to endemic infection, such as BVD, *Leptospira hardjo* and *Neospora caninum*. Heifers entering the herd, having been reared in isolation from the lactating cows, are susceptible and suffer a high rate of detectable loss, especially in the first year.

A similar pattern of loss was found in one of the herds we monitored in the course of studies at the Nottingham University School of Agriculture. BVD infection was present in the herd and was implicated as the cause. In two further herds in the study, high levels of loss were associated with clinical infections of IBR. In another herd there was a high rate of loss in cows inseminated naturally by a bull that was subsequently found to be infected with *Campylobacter fetus*. It has been shown that IBR and BVD viruses can infect the embryo or young fetus directly. Recent evidence has also shown that IBR and BVD can act at the ovarian level to compromise progesterone levels. In other cases of infection by these and other agents, the direct cause of the loss could be heat stress (resulting from infection-induced fever), which may damage the embryo at an early stage, with some deaths not occurring until some weeks later.

A wide number of infectious agents have been implicated in embryo and fetal death, including mycoplasma and salmonella, but a comprehensive study of these is beyond the scope of this book.

Insemination during pregnancy: milk progesterone studies at the National Institute for Research in Dairying, Reading, Nottingham University and SAC (Ball, 1997) revealed that more than 10% of inseminations in the herds under study were carried out at the wrong time (i.e., not within two days of an ovulation as detected by the profile). These included several inadvertent inseminations of pregnant cows. In about half of these cases, the existing conceptus was lost. In one instance, twin fetuses of approximately 30 days' gestation were seen to be aborted two days after insemination of a cow that was just over one month pregnant (see Fig. 12.8). This was in exact accordance with the information in the cow's milk progesterone profile. In other cases the fall in progesterone occurred up to at least a month after the mistimed insemination. The insemination may have caused infection or damage which ultimately killed the fetus, or the fetus may have died and been either resorbed or expelled after a delay, as discussed above under 'Incidence and timings of loss'.

The fact that in about half of the cases the conceptus survives and the cow gives birth to a calf from the original insemination suggests that many of the losses associated with incorrect insemination could be avoided by performing a 'cow-side' progesterone test and avoiding insemination if progesterone is present.

A simpler, but less efficient method would be to inseminate possibly pregnant cows halfway into the cervix rather than into the uterus. Weaver *et al.* (1989) deliberately re-inseminated cows into the uterine body, in the absence of oestrus, 12–24 days after a normal insemination at oestrus. These cows

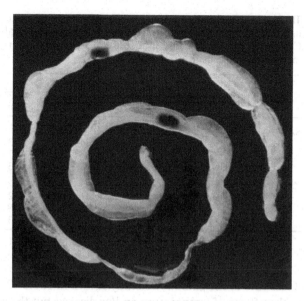

Fig. 12.8 Twin fetuses recovered from the vulval lips of a progesterone monitored cow after insemination during pregnancy.

had significantly lower pregnancy rates than controls that had not been re-inseminated (4% vs. 40.6%). Differences in pregnancy rates when the re-insemination was performed in the mid-cervical region were not statistically significant (34.8 vs. 50% for controls). They concluded that intrauterine insemination of cows displaying questionable signs of oestrus should be avoided in previously inseminated cows.

The problem might be due to herdsperson error in some cases; however, there are documented cases of cattle showing oestrus during pregnancy. It is worth repeating that a milk progesterone test would prevent mistimed insemination in such cases.

Ageing of ova: there is evidence (P.J.H. Ball, unpublished observations) that cows inseminated on the day after oestrus show a greater tendency to undergo embryonic mortality than those inseminated on the day of oestrus. This suggests that ageing ova are capable of being fertilized, but that some abnormality develops so that the resultant embryo is incapable of developing into a full-term fetus.

Ageing of cows: Ball (1978) reported a marked increase in the level of loss, as estimated from milk progesterone profiles, in older cows, particularly from the fifth lactation onwards. Subsequently, the same trend has been found in a number of studies, including those reported by Ball (1997) (see Table 12.7).

Table 12.7 Incidence of embryo fetal loss as estimated using milk progesterone profiles in Scottish Agricultural College (SAC) studies and in a study of large-scale commercial dairy herds in Zimbabwe.

	Lactation		
	1–5	*>5*	*Total*
SAC			
Conceptions	59	34	93
Losses	4	13	17
Percentage loss	6.8	38	18.3
Zimbabwe			
Conceptions	111	11	122
Losses	22	6	28
Percentage loss	19.8	55	23

The overall loss rate in the Zimbabwe study shown in Table 12.7 was higher, possibly due to the effects of temperature and/or disease, but the relative levels of loss were again significantly higher in older cows. This may have been due to the reduced ability of the uterus, having undergone a number of previous pregnancies, to support a subsequent implantation. Transfers of embryos from both young and old rabbits to the uteri of young rabbits resulted in good embryo survival whereas transfer from equivalent donors to the uteri of old rabbits resulted in reduced survival (Larson *et al.*, 1973). This suggested that the reduced reproductive efficiency of older does was due to the reduced ability of the aged uterus to support implantation, possibly due to reduced capacity for progesterone uptake, rather than to the reduced viability of ova from older ovaries. It could be speculated that the same was true for dairy cows. The cost of a comparable experiment using an adequate number of cows would be prohibitive.

Wiebold (1988) found that early embryonic mortality was associated with a uterine environment (as assessed by the composition of uterine flushings) significantly different from that of cows with normal embryos. Also, cows with an abnormal morula or blastocyst were significantly older and of greater parity than cows with an abnormal cleavage stage embryo. If the same were true at later stages after insemination, it would add weight to the idea that uterine, rather than embryo/fetal, deficiencies were responsible for the higher rate of loss in older cows. Plasma progesterone concentration did not differ between cows with normal embryos and those with abnormal embryos, or between cows with abnormal morulae or blastocysts and those with abnormal cleavage-stage embryos. However, it remains a possibility that the problem of later losses in older cows is due to reduced efficiency of progesterone production by their corpora lutea. This was not corroborated by Lamming *et al.* (1989), who found no differences in milk progesterone levels immediately preceding loss compared with cows at the same stage of pregnancy that did not suffer loss.

Prostaglandin administration: PGF$_{2\alpha}$ and its analogues can be 100% effective as abortive agents during the first few months of pregnancy in cattle. Any inadvertent injection of prostaglandin to a cow in the first trimester of pregnancy is therefore likely to cause pregnancy failure.

Pregnancy diagnosis (PD): rectal palpation, especially when performed earlier than about 55 days after insemination, has often been implicated in subsequent loss of the conceptus, but not all reports agree (see Ball, 1997). It is possible that PD by palpation could cause embryo death, but that minimal palpation may have no detrimental effect on survival. It is likely that using membrane slip and palpation of the amniotic vesicle in addition to fetal fluid fluctuation could cause more deaths than fetal fluid fluctuation alone.

Some clinicians feel that, to be effective, PD should be made by 50 days after insemination. However, this is less critical if some form of preliminary diagnosis (e.g., milk progesterone at around 21 days) has already been made, and in any case re-insemination would still not be carried out until about 63 days after the unsuccessful insemination unless prostaglandin was administered. Spontaneous loss is more likely up to about 60 days after insemination. The results of palpation after this time are thus more likely to give an accurate prediction of successful calvings, and in any case the procedure is far less risky than at 35–45 days of embryonic age.

There have been suggestions that PD by means of ultrasound scanning can lead to the death of the conceptus, but on balance the evidence suggests that this is not likely (see Ball, 1997).

Heat stress: high ambient temperatures, mediated by a rise in maternal body temperature, are known to affect conception rate and to cause the death of early bovine embryos, but there is less evidence of the deleterious effect of heat on the older conceptus. Studies have shown a reduction in progesterone level and/or corpus luteum size during pregnancy as a result of heat stress. This could in turn affect the viability of later embryos and fetuses. In general, it seems plausible that heat could damage the very early embryo, affecting its subsequent survival, so that a detectable loss occurs (see Ball, 1997).

Twin pregnancy: it might be expected that pregnancy in cattle would be compromised by the presence of two conceptuses, especially if both are implanting in the same uterine horn. Hanrahan (1983) concluded that the probability of embryo loss increased by 22% for unilateral compared with bilateral twin ovulations or single ovulations, but in general the evidence in the literature is inconclusive.

Early conception: west of Scotland milk progesterone studies showed a very clear relationship between days from calving to conception and subsequent embryo loss rates (Fig. 12.9). Conception rates were much lower and detectable loss rates much higher in cows inseminated earlier, especially before 50 days

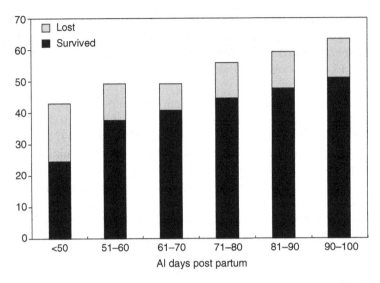

Fig. 12.9 Conception rate (in %) (full bars) and final pregnancy rate after detectable loss (in %) (solid bars) related to insemination (days postpartum).

postpartum. Only 43% of inseminations before 50 days postpartum resulted in conceptions capable of prolonging the life of the corpus luteum beyond 25 days, and 43% of these conceptions were subsequently lost.

This confirms an earlier report (Ball, 1980) that cows apparently suffering detectable loss had conceived sooner after the previous calving ($P < 0.001$) than cows maintaining a full-term pregnancy, suggesting that the problem was related to the environment in a uterus that had insufficient time to recover from the previous pregnancy and to be capable of supporting a subsequent implantation. Further confirmation of these findings was reported by Humblot (2001), who found that 17% of AIs before 70 days postpartum resulted in late embryonic mortality as compared to 13% of AIs more than 70 days postpartum. In practice, cows of high genetic merit and high predicted yield, as well as those with very low condition scores or with lameness and other problems, should be allowed longer delays to first service. Only in very exceptional circumstances should a cow be inseminated before 50 days and we suggest 60 days as a normal minimum.

Humblot (2001) has reviewed attempts to identify the environmental and genetic factors influencing early and/or late embryonic mortality in both temperate and subtropical environments.

Abortion

Abortion may be defined as the expulsion of a dead or non-viable fetus at any stage of pregnancy before the time of normal parturition. Normally the term is used for losses occurring after about the third month of pregnancy, when the expelled fetus is more likely to be seen by the herdsperson. A fetus is not always

Table 12.8 Causes of fetopathy (abortion) in cattle in the UK as diagnosed by the Veterinary Investigation Service. NR = not recorded. (From VIDA II, Veterinary Laboratories Agency, 2003.)

Cause	1983	1992	2001
Bovine viral diarrhoea (BVD)	82	140	34
Brucella abortus	50	0	0
Campylobacter spp	14	21	21
Corynebacterium (A) pyogenes	434	61	31
Leptospira spp	237	693	35
Listeria monocytogenes	29	23	18
Salmonella spp	282	221	92
Neospora	NR	NR	293
Fungi	227	96	38
Infectious bovine rhinotracheitis (IBR)	48	83	7
Other	323	127	71
No diagnosis	29 919	26 198	3123
Total	31 645	27 663	3763

aborted after it dies. Occasionally, its body fluids are reabsorbed by the cow and the fetus becomes 'mummified', in which case hormone therapy or even surgery are required to remove it. Sometimes, if the fetus has been killed by an infection it may degenerate within the uterus, so that again abortion does not occur.

If a dead calf is delivered after about 260 days of pregnancy when a normal calf would be capable of independent life outside the uterus, premature still-birth rather than abortion is said to have occurred. Most abortions are caused by infectious agents such as have already been discussed and this is why the problem is now much less common in developed countries in which diseases such as brucellosis have been controlled. Table 12.8 reports the diagnoses of the causes of abortion from material submitted to the UK Veterinary Investigation Service. The figures only give a general guide to the relative importance of the various pathogens since they depend on submission of aborted fetuses by farmers. The sharp drop in overall numbers in the latest ten years is partly accounted for by a fall in UK cow numbers and may largely be due to a fall in submission rates, rather than an improvement in abortion rates. Note the relatively high numbers of neospora infections and also the high level of undiagnosed abortions.

A variety of non-infectious factors can result in abortion. These include toxic agents such as nitrates, chlorinated naphthalene and some plant toxins. Physiological stress caused, for example, by severe fright or the trauma of being transported has been implicated in abortions probably because of glucocorticoid release. Nutritional problems leading to deficiencies of chemicals such as vitamin A, iodine and selenium may also cause or increase the likelihood of abortion. Abortion has also been reported to occur as a result of twin pregnancy.

References

Alt, D.P., Zuerner, R.L. & Bolin, C.A. (2001) *Journal of the American Veterinary Medical Association*, **219**, 636–639.

Arthur, G.H., Noakes, D.E., Pearson, H. & Parkinson, T.J. (1996) *Veterinary Reproduction and Obstetrics*, 7th edn. Baillière Tindall, London.

Ayalon, N. (1984) *Proceedings of the 10th International Congress on Animal Reproduction and Artificial Insemination*, **3**, 41. University of Illinois, Urbana.

Båge, R., Petyim, S., Larsson, B., Hallap, T., Bergqvist, A.S., Gustafsson, H. & Rodríguez-Martínez, H. (2003) *Reproduction Fertility and Development*, **15**, 115–123.

Ball, P.J.H. (1978) *Research in Veterinary Science*, **25**, 120–122.

Ball, P.J.H. (1980) *British Cattle Breeders Club Digest*, **35**, 54–58.

Ball, P.J.H. (1982) *British Veterinary Journal*, **138**, 546.

Ball, P.J.H. (1995) *Proceedings of the Nutec Dairy Workshop*, Lichfield, pp. 13–19.

Ball, P.J.H. (1997) *Animal Breeding Abstracts*, **65**, 167–175 (Review).

Ball, P.J.H. & McEwan, E.E.A. (1998) *Proceedings of the Annual Meeting of the British Society of Animal Science*, Scarborough, April, p. 187.

Bishop, M.W. (1964) *Journal of Reproduction and Fertility*, **7**, 383.

Biuk-Rudan, N., Cvetnić, S., Madić, J. & Rudan, D. (1999) *Theriogenology*, **51**, 875–881.

Block, S.S., Butler, W.R., Ehrhardt, R.A., Bell, A.W., Van Amburgh, M.E. & Boisclair, Y.R. (2001) *Journal of Endocrinology*, **171**, 339–348.

Boger, L.A. & Hattel, A.L. (2003) *Veterinary Parasitology*, **113**, 1–6.

Borsberry, S. & Dobson, H. (1989) *Veterinary Record*, **124**, 217–219.

BSAS (1995) *Proceedings of the British Society of Animal Science, Occasional Publication No. 19 – Breeding and Feeding the High Genetic Merit Dairy Cow*, Antrim, 1994.

Bulman, D.C. & Lamming, G.E. (1977) *Veterinary Record*, **100**, 550.

Carroll, E.J., Ball, L. & Scott, J.A. (1963) *Journal of the American Veterinary Medical Association*, **142**, 1105.

Charlier, C., Denys, B., Belanche, J.I., Coppieters, W., Grobet, L., Mni, M., Womack, J., Hanset, R. & Georges, M. (1996) *Mammalian Genome*, **7**, 138–142.

Collick, D.W., Ward, W.R. & Dobson, H. (1989) *Veterinary Record*, **125**, 103–106.

Crawshaw, W.M. & Brocklehurst, S. (2003) *Veterinary Record*, **152**, 201–206.

De Bois, C.H.W. (1982) In *Factors Influencing Fertility in the Post-Partum Cow* (eds H. Karg & E. Schallenberger), p. 479. Martinus Nijhoff, The Hague.

Dobson, H. & Smith, R.F. (2000) *Animal Reproduction Science*, **60–61**, 743–752.

Dobson, H., Ribadu, A.Y., Noble, K.M., Tebble, J.E. & Ward, W.R. (2000) *Journal of Reproduction and Fertility*, **120**, 405–410.

Douthwaite, R. & Dobson, H. (2000) *Veterinary Record*, **147**, 355–359.

Ennis, S., Vaughan, L. & Gallagher, T.F. (1999) *Research in Veterinary Science*, **67**, 111–112.

Frazier, K.S., Baldwin, C.A., Pence, M., West, J., Bernard, J., Liggett, A., Miller, D. & Hines, M.E. (2002) *Journal of Veterinary Diagnostic Investigation*, **14**, 457–462.

Gayerie, F. (1983) *Proceedings of the Society for the Study of Animal Breeding*.

Gerardi, A.S. (1996) *Research in Veterinary Science*, **61**, 183–186.

Gümen, A. & Seguin, B. (2003) *Theriogenology*, **60**, 341–348.

Hanrahan, J.P. (1983) *Theriogenology*, **20**, 3–11.

Heuwieser, W., Tenhagen, B.A., Tischer, M., Lühr, J. & Blum, H. (2000) *Veterinary Record*, **146**, 338–341.

Hickey, G.J., White, M.E., Wickenden, R.P. & Armstrong, D.A. (1984) *Veterinary Record*, **114**, 189.

Hockett, M.E., Hopkins, F.M., Lewis, M.J., Saxton, A.M., Dowlen, H.H., Oliver, S.P. & Schrick, F.N. (2000) *Animal Reproduction Science*, **58**, 241–251.

Hooijer, G.A., Lubbers, R.B., Ducro, B.J., van Arendonk, J.A., Kaal-Lansbergen, L.M. & van der Lende, T. (2001) *Journal of Dairy Science*, **84**, 286–291.

Humblot, P. (2001) *Theriogenology*, **56**, 1417–1433.

Huszenicza, G., Janosi, S., Kulcsar, M., Korodi, P., Dieleman, S.J., Bartyik, J., Rudas, P. & Ribiczei-Szabo, P. (1998) *Reproduction in Domestic Animals*, **33**, 147–153.

Jánosa, A., Baranyai, B. & Dohy, J. (1999) *Acta Veterinarica Hungarica*, **47**, 283–289.

Kastelic, J.P., Northey, D.L. & Ginther, O.J. (1991) *Theriogenology*, **35**, 351–363.

Königsson, K., Gustafsson, H., Gunnarsson, A. & Kindahl, H. (2001) *Reproduction in Domestic Animals*, **36**, 247–256.

Kruip, T.A.M., Wensing, T. & Vos, P.L.A.M. (2001) In *Fertility in the High-Producing Dairy Cow* (ed. M. Diskin), *British Society of Animal Science Occasional Publication*, **26**, 63–79.

Lamming, G.E., Darwash, A.O. & Back, H.L. (1989) *Journal of Reproduction and Fertility*, Suppl. **37**, 245–252.

Larson, L.L., Spilman, C.H. & Dunn, H.O. (1973) *Journal of Reproduction and Fertility*, **33**, 31–38.

Laven, R.A. & Peters, A.R. (1996) *Veterinary Record*, **139**, 465–471.

Laven, R.A., Biggadike, H.J. & Allison, R.D. (2002) *Reproduction in Domestic Animals*, **37**, 111–115.

LeBlanc, S.J., Duffield, T.F., Leslie, K.E., Bateman, K.G., Keefe, G.P., Walton, J.S. & Johnson, W.H. (2002a) *Journal of Dairy Science*, **85**, 2223–2236.

LeBlanc, S.J., Duffield, T.F., Leslie, K.E., Bateman, K.G., Keefe, G.P., Walton, J.S. & Johnson, W.H. (2002b) *Journal of Dairy Science*, **85**, 2237–2249.

López-Gatius, F., Santolaria, P., Yániz, J., Rutllant, J. & López-Béjar, M. (2001) *Theriogenology*, **56**, 649–659.

Makoschey, B. & Keil, G.M. (2000) *Veterinary Record*, **147**, 189–191.

Maley, S.W., Buxton, D., Rae, A.G., Wright, S.E., Schock, A., Bartley, P.M., Esteban-Redondo, I., Swales, C., Hamilton, C.M., Sales, J. & Innes, E.A. (2003) *Journal of Comparative Pathology*, **129**, 186–195.

Mann, G.E. & Lamming, G.E. (1999) *Reproduction in Domestic Animals*, **34**, 269–274.

Marshall, J.F., Barrett, D.C., Logue, D.N., Ball, P.J.H. & Mihm, M. (2003) *Cattle Practice*, **11**, 151–152.

Maurer, R.R. & Echternkamp, S.E. (1985) *Journal of Animal Science*, **61**, 624.

McClure, T.J. (1994) *Nutritional and Metabolic Infertility in the Cow*. CAB International, Wallingford.

Miller, R., Chelmonska-Soyta, A., Smits, B., Foster, R. & Rosendal, S. (1994) *Veterinary Clinics of North America–Food Animal Practice*, **10**, 479–490.

Mizushima, S. & Fukui, Y. (2001) *Theriogenology*, **55**, 1431–1445.

MLC (1981) *Beef Production Yearbook*.

Panangala, V.S., Winter, A.J., Wijesinha, A. & Foote, R.H. (1981) *American Journal of Veterinary Research*, **42**, 2090–2093.

Parkinson, T.J., Smith, K.C., Long, S.E., Douthwaite, J.A., Mann, G.E. & Knight, P.G. (2001) *Reproduction*, **122**, 397–409.

Peters, A.R. (1996) *Animal Breeding Abstracts*, **64**, 587–598.

Peters, A.R. & Laven, R.A. (1996) *Veterinary Record*, **139**, 535–539.

Peeler, E.J., Otte, M. & Esslemont, R.J. (1994) *Veterinary Record*, **134**, 129–132.

Peters, A.R., Martinez, T.A. & Cook, A.J. (2000) *Theriogenology*, **54**, 1317–1326.

Ragan, V.E. (2002) *Veterinary Microbiology*, **90**, 11–18.

Reist, M., Erdin, D.K., von Euw, D., Tschümperlin, K.M., Leuenberger, H., Hammon, H.M., Künzi, N. & Blum, J.W. (2003) *American Journal of Veterinary Research*, **64**, 188–194.

Rota, A., Ballarin, C., Vigier, B., Cozzi, B. & Rey, R. (2002) *General and Comparative Endocrinology*, **129**, 39–44.

Saacke, R.G., Dalton, J.C., Nadir, S., Nebel, R.L. & Bame, J.H. (2000) *Animal Reproduction Science*, **60–61**, 663–677.

Sanderson, M.W., Chenoweth, P.J., Yeary, T. & Nietfeld, J.C. (2000) *Theriogenology*, **54**, 401–408.

Satoh, S., Hirata, T. & Miyake, Y. (1997) *Journal of Veterinary Medical Science*, **59**, 221–222.

Schurig, G.G., Sriranganathan, N. & Corbel, M.J. (2002) *Veterinary Microbiology*, **90**, 479–496.

Sheldon, I.M., Noakes, D.E., Rycroft, A.N., Pfeiffer, D.U. & Dobson, H. (2002) *Reproduction*, **123**, 837–845.

Silvia, W.J., Hatler, T.B., Nugent, A.M. & Laranja da Fonseca, L.F. (2002) *Domestic Animal Endocrinology*, **23**, 167–177.

Smith, R.F., Gore, S.W., Phogat, P.B. & Dobson, H. (1997) *Journal of Endocrinology*, **152** (Suppl. P172).

Stables, J.W. (1980) *The Bovine Practitioner*, **15**, 26.

Starbuck, G.R., Gutierrez, C.G. & Mann, G.E. (2000) *Journal of Reproduction and Fertility Abstract Series*, **25**, Abstract 55.

Starbuck, G.R., Darwash, A.O., Mann, G.E. & Lamming, G.E. (2001) In *Fertility in the High-Producing Dairy Cow* (ed. M. Diskin), *British Society of Animal Science Occasional Publication*, **26**, 447–450.

Taylor, V.J., Beever, D.E., Bryant, M.J. & Wathes, D.C. (2003) *Theriogenology*, **59**, 1661–1677.

Tefera, N., Jeanguyot, N., Thibier, M. & Humblot, P. (2001) *Journal of Veterinary Medicine Series A–Physiology Pathology Clinical Medicine*, **48**, 331–336.

Thompson, J.G. & Peterson, A.J. (2000) *Human Reproduction*, **15** (Suppl. 5), 59–67.

Van Drunen Littel-van den Hurk, S., Myers, D., Doig, P.A., Karvonen, B., Habermehl, M., Babiuk, L.A., Jelinski, M., Van Donkersgoed, J., Schlesinger, K. & Rinehart, C. (2001) *Canadian Journal of Veterinary Research*, **65**, 81–88.

Veterinary Laboratories Agency (2003) *Veterinary Investigation Surveillance Report II.* VLA, Weighbridge.

Waldner, C.L., Janzen, E.D. & Henderson, J. (1999) *Journal of the American Veterinary Medical Association*, **215**, 1485–1490.

Wathes, D.C., Taylor, V.J., Cheng, Z. & Mann, G.E. (2003) *Reproduction* (Suppl. 61), 219–237.

Weaver, L.D., Daley, C.A. & Borelli, C.L. (1989) *Theriogenology*, **32**, 603–606.

Wiebold, J.L. (1988) *Journal of Reproduction and Fertility*, **84**, 393–399.

Wolfenson, D., Roth, Z. & Meidan, R. (2000) *Animal Reproduction Science*, **60–61**, 535–547.

Chapter 13
Reproductive Biotechnologies

Many examples of biotechnology, in its broadest sense, are already in use as aids to cattle reproductive management and have been referred to in previous chapters. These include the technologies associated with oestrus detection, oestrous cycle control and artificial insemination. This chapter is intended to give a brief introduction to technologies that are not covered, or mentioned only briefly, elsewhere. In most instances, it is not intended that this chapter should give a complete and detailed coverage of the procedures and their uses, and the reader is referred to appropriate references for this purpose.

Reproductive monitoring

Automatic progesterone measurement

Milk progesterone measurement can be an extremely useful tool to aid reproductive management. Its use in the detection of ovulation (Chapter 8) and for pregnancy diagnosis (Chapter 11) have been discussed. The ability to measure individual cow milk progesterone levels automatically during milking would considerably improve the usefulness of the technique in some situations. A number of scientists have attempted to develop methods that fulfil such requirements. At the time of writing, none have yet been developed sufficiently to be of commercial use, but some show promise. Pemberton *et al.* (2001) have developed an electrochemical biosensor in which anti-progesterone monoclonal antibody is deposited onto screen-printed carbon electrodes. Progesterone in the sample to be measured competes with alkaline-phosphatase-labelled progesterone for binding sites on the electrode. As with manual enzyme-based assays, the more progesterone in the sample, the less 'labelled' progesterone binds to the antibody. The amount of bound, labelled progesterone is estimated by establishing a baseline electric current and measuring the extent to which this is altered in the presence of an enzyme substrate.

Another method that shows some promise, and avoids the need for an enzyme label, was reported by Gillis *et al.* (2002). A sensor surface is prepared by covalently immobilizing progesterone to a carboxymethyl dextran matrix on a chip. A fixed amount of antiprogesterone monoclonal antibody is mixed with the sample in a constant ratio and injected over the sensor surface. Resultant changes in the refractive index of the solution close to the sensor are used to estimate progesterone levels in the sample. The procedure involves fully automated instrumentation and has potential to be used in-line during milking.

Other methods, which seem to show less promise, include measurement of change in the oscillating frequency of an antibody-coated crystal in response to the amount of progesterone bound to it (Koelsch *et al.*, 1994) and an automated ELISA test (Claycomb *et al.*, 1995).

Automatic detection of oestrus-related chemicals

There has been considerable interest in the development of a so-called Electronic Nose – an automated device which can detect olfactory signals electronically. Since Kiddy *et al.* (1978) demonstrated that dogs could be trained to detect odours associated with cows in oestrus it has been apparent that they secrete pheromonal chemicals which could be potentially measured electronically. Mottram *et al.* (2000) developed and evaluated a potential method of oestrus detection. It consisted of conducting polymer sensors and a system for sampling, humidity management and data analysis. The most reliable results were obtained when swabs were obtained from the cervical area and placed in a sample chamber. This is not easily applicable to practical oestrus detection, although it may have potential for the confirmation of oestrus in some circumstances. The authors concluded that immunosensor technology such as that being developed for automatic progesterone measurement appeared to be the most appropriate method of predicting ovulation.

Sex determination

There are areas in which cattle management could be improved if calves of a predetermined sex could be produced. Dairy farmers, for example, would prefer most of their calves to be female and thus potentially become replacements for the milking herd. Most Holstein male beef calves have a very low value in many countries. Faster genetic gain can be expected, especially if the technique is used in conjunction with schemes such as MOET (multiple ovulation and embryo transfer). Beef farmers may often prefer their cows to produce bull calves, although the economic advantage may be less pronounced. There are two main approaches to producing a calf of a particular sex: (1) determination of the gender of embryos and selecting those of the desired sex for transfer, and (2) using either X- or Y-bearing spermatozoa to produce female or male embryos respectively.

Embryo sexing

A number of methods have been used with some degree of success to determine the sex of an embryo before it is transferred to a recipient. These include:

- Karyotyping. Individual cells are removed from the embryo, usually without compromising its viability, and checked to see if they are XX (female) or XY (male) (Winterberger-Torres & Popescu, 1980).

- Immunology. Antibodies are used to detect the presence of male-specific antigens (White & Anderson, 1987; Utsumi & Iritani, 1993).
- Detection of metabolic differences (Rieger, 1984), including the colorimetric assay of an enzyme linked to the X chromosome (Williams, 1986).
- DNA analysis (Bredbacka *et al.*, 1995). This approach has been facilitated by the use of polymerase chain reaction to amplify specific stretches of DNA, such that the technique is now available commercially (Shea, 1999).

The main drawback to embryo sexing is that embryos of the unwanted sex are usually discarded, resulting in a waste of resources.

Semen sexing

If semen were sexed, embryos of the required sex could be produced, either in vivo or in vitro, thus avoiding the effort and wastage of having to determine the sex of an embryo, and then possibly discarding it if it proves to be of the wrong gender. Sexed semen is potentially of use (1) in practical management to inseminate cows with the aim of producing calves of the required sex and (2) for the fertilization of oocytes in vitro to produce embryos of the required sex.

For many decades there have been attempts to separate X- and Y-bearing spermatozoa on the basis of their physical, biological and immunological properties. The latter has shown some promise, with the possibility that sex-specific antigens could be present on bovine spermatozoa (Howes *et al.*, 1997). The ultimate aim would be to immunize mice with the appropriate protein, use individual immune cells to produce antibody in tissue culture and to grow the best cultures on an industrial scale to produce pure monoclonal antibody. The appropriate antibody would then be used to kill spermatozoa of the unwanted type. The existence and siting of such antigens is still not well established, and this and other procedures have been overtaken by the development of flow cytometry techniques, whose use has been reviewed by Seidel (2003).

Flow cytometry is made possible by the fact that X-bearing sperm contains 3–4% more DNA than Y-bearing sperm and the availability of a fluorescent dye which binds specifically to nucleic acids. Details can be found in the literature (e.g., Seidel, 2002) and only a simple overview of the procedures used will be provided here:

- Freshly collected semen is stored undiluted for up to 9 hours.
- Aliquots of semen are stained with a fluorescent dye (Hoechst 33342) which permeates the cell membrane and binds specifically to adenine–thymine base pairs on the DNA molecules of the chromosomes. Female spermatozoa would be expected to take up more dye.
- Sperm are diluted in a sorting medium.

- Spermatozoa in the sorting medium are introduced into a flow cytometer within a cylindrical wall of sheath fluid, which guides the flow of liquid through the sorter.
- An oscillating crystal divides the liquid flow into droplets containing individual spermatozoa.
- As each spermatozoon passes a pair of detectors a laser beam causes fluorescence of the dye, and the detectors measure the intensity of fluorescence so that a computer can determine whether it is X or Y bearing.
- A positive or negative charge is applied to each droplet according to whether the spermatozoon in it is X or Y bearing. Droplets failing to meet the determined criteria are not charged.
- The droplets pass between a pair of continuously charged plates, which attract oppositely charged particles, deflecting the flow towards a receptacle for the appropriate type of sperm. Uncharged droplets pass undeflected into a waste container.

The process is illustrated in Fig. 13.1 and components of the equipment used are shown in Fig. 13.2.

The percentage of sperm in the original ejaculate that actually survive the sorting and subsequent freezing process is, not surprisingly, very low. However, the final sample contains a very high proportion of healthy, viable spermatozoa so that, using techniques such as 'multi thermal gradient' freezing (Chapter 10), it has been possible to use sexed semen for live cow insemination as well as for in vitro fertilization. The sale of sexed bovine sperm commenced in the UK in September 2000.

Embryo transfer

Almost a century has elapsed since the first successful mammalian embryo transfer was achieved by Heape (1890) in the rabbit. In 1951 Willett *et al.* completed the first viable bovine embryo transfer, and in 1964 Mutter *et al.* reported an isolated success with the non-surgical transfer of an embryo between cows. Embryo transfer work in cattle has always tended to lag behind that in many other species and real progress in cattle embryo transfer did not take place until the late 1960s and early 1970s. This progress was largely as the result of work by Rowson and colleagues at Cambridge (Rowson *et al.*, 1969).

Experience and techniques have developed to the extent that embryo transfer is now a commercial proposition in many countries throughout the world and is widespread in countries such as the USA, Canada and Australia.

Embryo transfer began in the UK on a significant scale in 1972. By the mid- to late 1980s it was estimated that there were 10 000 embryo transfers per year in Great Britain, although the outbreaks of BSE and foot-and-mouth disease at the turn of the century will have led to a subsequent lowering of this figure.

The main reason for the development of embryo transfer in cattle was to further the increase in genetic progress made possible by the adoption of AI.

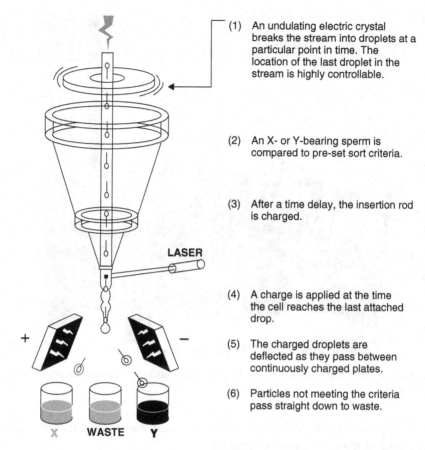

(1) An undulating electric crystal breaks the stream into droplets at a particular point in time. The location of the last droplet in the stream is highly controllable.

(2) An X- or Y-bearing sperm is compared to pre-set sort criteria.

(3) After a time delay, the insertion rod is charged.

LASER

(4) A charge is applied at the time the cell reaches the last attached drop.

(5) The charged droplets are deflected as they pass between continuously charged plates.

(6) Particles not meeting the criteria pass straight down to waste.

X   WASTE   Y

Fig. 13.1 X and Y sperm separation by flow cytometry. (Courtesy of Cogent.)

In particular, it can be used to create large families of contemporary full siblings, which can be used for sibling testing as used in MOET (multiple ovulation embryo transfer) schemes. Very high genetic merit males and females are identified, the females are superovulated and inseminated, and the embryos are then transferred to individual recipient females. The resulting full sibling families are, when mature, available for testing.

Embryo transfer offers a means of transporting livestock between countries at less expense and without the trauma associated with the transport of adult animals. Animals transported as embryos and developing within recipients in the destination country are likely to adapt more readily to local conditions than those transported as adults. Apart from genetic improvement within breeds, embryo transport offers a convenient means of introducing new breeds where they may be of benefit. For example, a herd of Red Dane cattle in Zimbabwe, resulting from the import of embryos, offers the potential of providing crosses

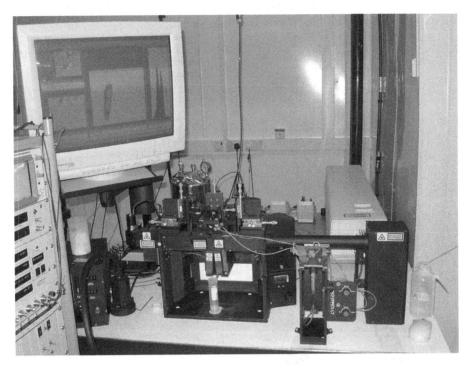

Fig. 13.2   Equipment used for X and Y sperm separation by flow cytometry. (Courtesy of Cogent.)

with indigenous cattle which would perform well under the harsh conditions pertaining in many areas of the country.

Other uses of embryo transfer include obtaining fertilized embryos from superior old cows that can no longer breed normally, although as a general rule better genetic progress could be expected from concentrating on younger stock.

Other techniques of reproductive manipulation, referred to later in this chapter, have embryo transfer as their basis. The technique is also a valuable research tool in the field of cattle reproductive physiology.

Embryo transfer procedures

Preparation of donor animals

It is quite feasible to collect single embryos from a donor animal after natural ovulation. However, in order to make the best use of the donor's potential and to maximize the return on the time and expense involved, it is normal to superovulate the cow so that a number of embryos can be collected from her at each flushing. At the same time, her oestrus/ovulation date may be induced to ensure synchrony with the recipient if fresh embryos are to be transferred.

Superovulation is induced by administering exogenous doses of hormones that have follicle stimulating hormone (FSH) activity to overcome the natural mechanism that would normally only allow one follicle to become dominant and ovulate. Pituitary extracts of bovine FSH have been used to induce super-ovulation particularly in the USA. However, since the half-life of FSH in the circulation is relatively short, repeated injections are required, usually over a five-day period. A crude horse anterior pituitary extract (HAP) has also been used successfully, but most superovulation in preparation for embryo transfer is induced using pregnant mare's serum gonadotrophin (PMSG) which has been found to have both FSH-like and LH-like properties, but has a much longer half life in the body (in excess of 50 hours as compared to approximately 0.5–1 hour for endogenous LH and FSH). There was concern in the early days of embryo transfer that repeated superovulation using PMSG might stimulate antibody production to the gonadotrophin, eventually rendering it ineffective. There was evidence that cows were becoming refractory to the hormone after repeated doses. These fears, however, do not seem to have been borne out by more recent experience.

The response of individual cows to PMSG is highly variable, but is to some extent dose-dependent. The number of ovulations produced normally ranges from one to well over 20. When large numbers of ovulations are induced the recovery of ova is less efficient, perhaps because their passage into the fimbria after ovulation is impaired. The proportion of normal fertilized eggs is also reduced. The usual dose is between 1500 and 3000 international units (IU) given as an intramuscular injection in a small volume of saline.

It is known that the presence of a dominant follicle can disrupt superovulatory response in cattle. McEvoy *et al.* (1996) showed that destruction of the dominant follicle by trans-vaginal aspiration of its contents (as used in ovum pick-up – see below) enhanced ovulation rates and yields of viable embryos. Merton *et al.* (2003), however, reported that the technique was advantageous in cows, but not in heifers.

The injection should be timed to coincide with luteolysis. This may be achieved by choosing the appropriate stage of the natural ovarian cycle, but it is preferable to control the cycle using either progestogens or prostaglandins so that the timing of ovulation can be controlled and predicted more closely. A typical regimen as used in preparing donors in the UK is as follows:

- PMSG is given at approximately 0900 hours one morning between days 9 and 12 of the cow's natural cycle.
- Ovulation is induced at a predetermined time by the injection of prostaglandin or an analogue to cause luteolysis. In practice, 2 mg of cloprostenol is injected at 0900 hours 2–3 days after the PMSG injection.
- The cloprostenol is followed 1.5 hours later by 250 mg of GnRH to ensure a good, well synchronized pre-ovulatory LH peak. The cow is expected to come into heat within a 24- to 96-hour period.

- Artificial insemination is carried out on the day of oestrus at 0900 hours using one 2.5-ml straw of semen. Between 1600 and 1700 hours on the same day a second insemination is carried out using two straws of semen. If the cow is still in oestrus at 2100 hours, a further insemination using one straw is carried out at 0900 hours on the next day.

Sreenan (1983) reported that at least 95% of cows thus treated showed oestrus after prostaglandin. Most authors report mean ovulation rates of between 8 and 18 ovulations and a fertilization rate of recovered eggs of around 80%.

Collection of embryos

Until the mid-1970s most successful embryo recoveries were carried out by means of surgery under general anaesthetic. Non-surgical collection via the cervix generally results in the recovery of around 10% fewer embryos, but is cheaper and simpler, avoids the risks of general anaesthesia and can be carried out on farms. Thus, most commercial embryo recoveries are now carried out non-surgically. Recovery via the cervix is only possible after the embryos have entered the uterus, and is thus normally carried out at or soon after day 6 of the oestrous cycle following superovulation.

The donor cow is restrained in a normal cattle crush, usually with her front feet higher than her hind feet to render the tract more accessible. The cow is usually tranquillized and given an epidural anaesthetic injection, after which embryos are flushed from the uterus using a Foley three-way catheter as shown in Fig. 13.3.

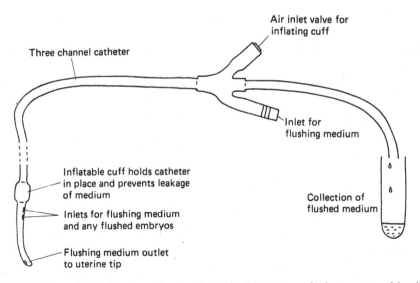

Fig. 13.3 Use of a Foley three-way catheter in the non-surgical recovery of bovine embryos.

The catheter has three channels: one for the admission of air to inflate a collar near the tip, one with an outlet very close to the tip for the entry of flushing medium and one with an opening slightly further from the tip for the collection of flushing media, plus any recovered embryos, from the uterus. The sterile catheter is inserted into the first uterine horn to be flushed (usually ipsilateral to the ovary which appears to have shed most ova), being protected from contamination in the vulva and vagina by means of sleeves which do not pass through the cervix. Once the catheter is in position, the collar is inflated by means of a syringe filled with air (Fig. 13.4a); this serves to hold the catheter in position and to prevent the leakage of flushing medium into the body of the uterus. A large volume of flushing medium (200–500 ml depending on the size of the cow or heifer) is injected by means of a syringe into the first channel and allowed to flow back through the outlet channel into a large test tube or glass cylinder, hopefully carrying a high proportion of embryos with it (Fig. 13.4b).

The catheter is then repositioned in the other uterine horn so that it may be flushed in the same way. The whole operation is facilitated by manipulation of the reproductive tract per rectum. Commercially available Dulbecco's PBS (phosphate buffered saline) ova culture medium, to which is added 4 mg per cent of bovine albumin, is used for flushing the tract and also for subsequent short-term storage and transfer of embryos. Embryos are slightly denser than the culture medium and thus tend to sink to the bottom of the collecting vessel, usually within two minutes. In practice, the collection vessels are allowed to stand for 10 minutes, after which it has been found that 98% of the embryos in the medium will be recovered. Most of the medium can be siphoned off after the embryos have settled so that they may be expected to be found in the remaining 10–20 ml. The embryos are just visible as small specks to the naked eye and can be seen and manipulated in small quantities of medium in glass Petri dishes under a low-power microscope (Fig. 13.5).

Storage of embryos

If embryos are to be transferred to recipient cows or heifers on the same day they may be stored in a fresh, sterile solution of the same culture medium for several hours, provided they are maintained close to body temperature. It is now possible to freeze cattle embryos for long-term storage, after which pregnancy rates in excess of 50% can be expected under the best conditions. The problems involved with freezing embryos are analogous to those of freezing semen, except that embryos are more sensitive to the freezing and thawing process and high wastage rates cannot be tolerated. As with spermatozoa, glycerol is often used as a cryoprotective agent. Embryos are normally stored individually in 0.25-ml straws such as are used for AI (Fig. 13.6) and are then reduced to liquid nitrogen temperature at a controlled rate.

After storage the embryos must be returned to body temperature at a controlled rate related to the speed at which they were originally cooled. For

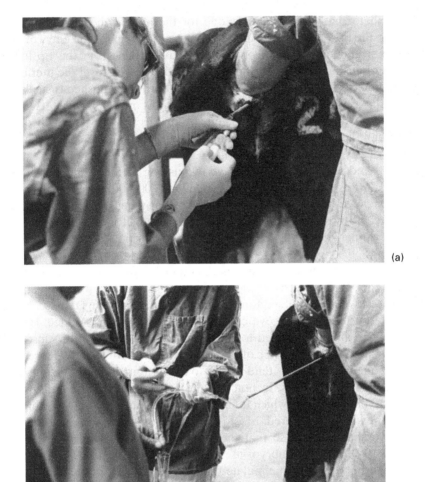

(a)

(b)

Fig. 13.4 Non-surgical collection of embryos: (a) inflation of collar; (b) flushing. (Courtesy of Mr R. Newcomb, and Mr W. Davies, Uzmaston Farm, Pembrokeshire.)

example, if they were cooled quickly there are likely to be small ice crystals within the embryonic cells. These embryos must then be warmed quickly so that the crystals thaw before they have a chance to enlarge and damage the cells. In practice the straws are thawed in 37°C water baths. Cryoprotectant then needs to be removed. This is carried out in stages to avoid osmotic shock.

More recently, simplified methods of cryopreservation have been developed (see Boland *et al.*, 2000). These include a one-step method, direct transfer after thawing, vitrification and ultra-rapid freezing. In the open pulled straw method (Vajta *et al.*, 1998) French mini-straws are heat softened and stretched to reduce

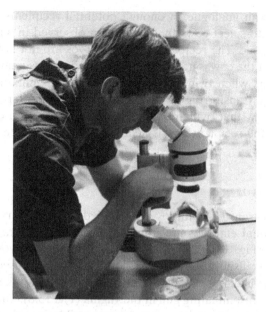

Fig. 13.5 Examination of medium for the presence of embryos. (Courtesy of Mr R. Newcomb.)

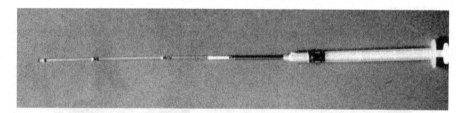

Fig. 13.6 Embryo prepared for storage or transfer. The embryo is in the central column of medium flanked by two air bubbles and two further columns of medium. Contents of straw are sucked in from the right, so that the first column of liquid moistens the cotton plug and forms a seal.

their diameter and wall thickness. Embryos are loaded by capillary action and vitrified by plunging the narrow end of the straw into liquid nitrogen. The very high rates of cooling and thawing thus achieved allow reduced exposure times to high concentrations of cryoprotectant.

Preparation of recipients

Embryo transfer has the greatest chance of success if the recipient animal is at the same day of her cycle as the donor on the day her eggs were collected. For the immediate transfer of fresh embryos, this means that donor and recipient should have been in oestrus on the same day, or within a day of each other. This can be achieved by synchronizing the recipient with an injection of prostaglandin or an analogue. If enough potential recipients are available it may be possible to select cows that have been observed in natural oestrus at the appropriate time. The recipient's own embryos are not normally required to develop so that the cow is neither superovulated nor inseminated. An exception to this occurs when twinning is attempted by inseminating the recipient and subsequently transferring another embryo into the uterine horn contralateral to the ovary that ovulated. The chances of success in embryo transfer are improved if the recipient cow is healthy, well fed and free from reproductive abnormalities.

Transfer of embryos

For non-surgical transfer, embryos are handled in plastic straws as shown in Fig. 13.6. Individual embryos are usually drawn into the straws by means of a small syringe (Fig. 13.7). Non-surgical transfer of embryos is carried out through the cervix, using a longer version of the apparatus used for AI. A very similar technique is employed, except that greater care is taken to avoid contamination of the inseminating gun in the vagina (Fig. 13.8). The embryo is also deposited further into the uterus – as far as possible into the horn ipsilateral to the ovary that ovulated.

Limitations

An average of five embryos per flush can be expected using non-surgical recovery methods, leading to an average of 50 freezable embryos per donor per year

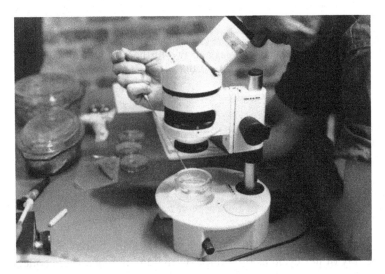

Fig. 13.7   Drawing the embryo into the straw in preparation for transfer. (Courtesy of Mr R. Newcomb.)

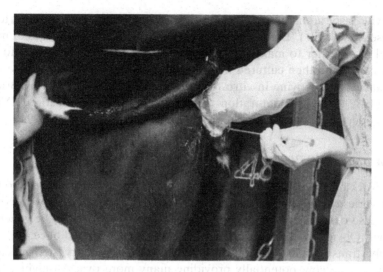

Fig. 13.8   Non-surgical embryo transfer. (Courtesy of Mr R. Newcomb.)

and the birth of around 30 calves (Merton *et al.*, 2003). About half of these could be of lesser value because they are of the wrong sex. In order to make the best use of MOET, it is necessary to minimize the generation interval. For example, performance testing can identify superior Simmental heifers by the time they are 11 months old. In order to maintain a two-year calving interval and provide for further selection in the next generation, multiple pregnancies must be established before the selected heifers are 15 months old, allowing very little time to obtain the target of 15 transferable embryos (McEvoy & Sinclair, 1997). Overall, embryo transfer has failed to achieve the increased rates of genetic progress that had been predicted.

In vitro embryo production

As was seen in Chapters 2 and 4, the ovary, from birth, contains a huge supply of ovum-containing follicles, groups (or cohorts) of which migrate to the surface and start to develop at regular seven- or ten-day intervals. The vast majority of these become atretic, but they do represent a potential source of ova for embryo production. If ova are harvested directly from the ovary (as opposed to collecting fertilized embryos from the uterus), there is potential to collect larger numbers more frequently and from younger cows.

   In vitro embryo production also offers the possibility of scientific investigation of conception- and pregnancy-related problems. Båge *et al.* (2003), for example, used the technique to establish that repeat breeder heifers also demonstrated deviation from controls in the production and subsequent in vitro development of oocytes. The procedure also plays a vital part in the production of transgenic animals (see below).

In vivo aspiration of oocytes via the vaginal wall was first reported by Pieterse *et al.* (1991). The oocytes collected will be at various stages of maturity and so, in order to make use of them, they need to be matured and fertilized in vitro and then cultured before final transfer to a recipient. Successful pregnancies from bovine in vitro fertilization were first reported by Brackett *et al.* (1982). In vitro maturation (IVM) and in vitro fertilization (IVF) of bovine oocytes is now a practical proposition (see, e.g., Gordon, 1994).

Ovum pickup (OPU)

Early work on in vitro embryo production involved the aspiration of oocytes from ovaries removed from cattle after slaughter. There were, however, inherent disease risks and the slaughtered cattle would not normally be genetically superior. Obviously, it is only possible to harvest each animal once.

Using transvaginal ovum pickup (OPU) ova can be harvested repeatedly from the same cow, potentially providing many more ova. An eight-year-old cow has produced 176 embryos during 158 weekly collections. Twice weekly aspiration may be better than weekly as it is more likely to pre-empt the development of a dominant follicle that could have a negative effect on results. Goodhand *et al.* (1999) found that twice- versus once-weekly aspiration doubled the number of transferable embryos produced per week. Båge *et al.* (2003) reported no depletion of follicles over time in spite of an intensive collection regimen involving 11–19 collection sessions during three to six oestrous cycles. Others, however, have shown decreased yields (but no loss of quality) with repeated collections. Provided that collections are timed to coincide with the naturally occurring development of follicular waves, these increased numbers of oocytes can be obtained without the need for superovulatory hormone treatments. Nevertheless, FSH treatment three days prior to aspiration can be beneficial. Goodhand *et al.* (1999) reported that the weekly transferable embryo yield from weekly aspirations was doubled as a result of FSH treatment and was similar to the weekly yield from twice weekly collection without FSH treatment. Roth *et al.* (2002) found that both BST pretreatment improved oocyte morphology and FSH pre-treatment improved morphology and cleavage rate, thus helping to overcome the effects of summer heat stress on oocytes harvested in the autumn.

A further advantage of OPU is that it can be performed during the first trimester of pregnancy and also on prepubertal, including fetal, animals. Results are generally worse and more variable in pre-pubertal, as opposed to adult, cattle, but there is potential for substantial improvement in genetic gain by markedly reducing the generation interval. Cows over 14 years of age yield fewer oocytes. These findings have been reviewed by Boland *et al.* (2000) and see also the detailed review of factors affecting oocyte quality and quantity by Merton *et al.* (2003).

The equipment used consists of an ultrasound apparatus whose transducer has a built-in needle guide. After epidural anaesthesia of the donor, the transducer is introduced into the vagina and the ovary to be aspirated is moved per rectum to a position just anterior to the vaginal fornix. Thus, follicles can be imaged and the needle guide used to pass an echogenic needle through the vaginal wall into the ovary. Target follicles are positioned and aspirated by means of a foot-controlled vacuum. The level of vacuum used represents a compromise between the need to retrieve the oocyte and at the same time maintaining the integrity of its surrounding cumulus cells (Boland *et al.*, 2000; McEvoy *et al.*, 2002). Fig. 13.9 illustrates an example of such equipment.

Questions have been raised about possible adverse physiological and/or welfare consequences for cows subjected to repeated OPU. McEvoy *et al.* (2002) concluded that ovarian function was not compromised after 13–16 aspirations, and that after 16–20 collections there was no evidence of infection or inflammation at the site of the epidural anaesthetic injection associated with OPU. Some minor damage was thought to be associated with imperfect procedures, rather than frequency of injection. Chastant-Maillard *et al.* (2003) studied stress-related physiological parameters (cortisol levels; adrenal sensitivity; blood and milk somatic cell counts), milk yields, ovarian function and morphology in cows during and after repeated OPU. The cows were compared with controls, which were handled and given epidural injection, but not subjected to vaginal puncture. They found no adverse welfare consequences of the OPU procedure per se.

In vitro maturation

One of the main drawbacks of in vitro embryo production is that less than 40% of oocytes obtained by OPU subsequently develop into blastocysts, probably because of the quality of the oocytes themselves, rather than the efficiency of subsequent procedures. This is hardly surprising when it is considered that a very high proportion of ovarian follicles are destined by nature to become atretic. Furthermore, the oocytes obtained will be at varying stages of development. Usually, they are obtained from follicles 2–8 mm in diameter. Without intervention such oocytes, if they are destined to ovulate, would have taken several more weeks to mature. Aspirated oocytes are matured for only 24 hours in vitro, during which time the same maturation processes need to take place. Various attempts and means of arresting the oocyte at the immature germinal vesicle stage have been reported (Boland *et al.*, 2000). It is thought that this may allow them the opportunity to acquire greater developmental competence before they are submitted to normal in vitro maturation. The presence of cumulous cells seems to be critical, especially in the early stages of maturation.

Cryopreservation of oocytes is possible, but it is much less successful than freezing embryos (see Boland *et al.*, 2000).

In vitro fertilization

Fertilization is effected by exposing the matured oocyte to capacitated spermatozoa, either fresh or frozen–thawed in a fertilization medium. Heparin is usually added to the medium to induce capacitation of the sperm. Mendes

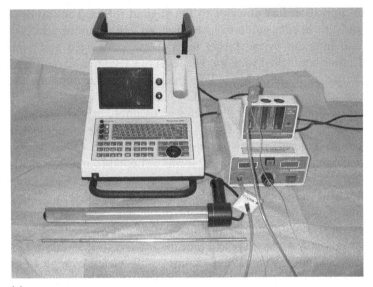

(a)

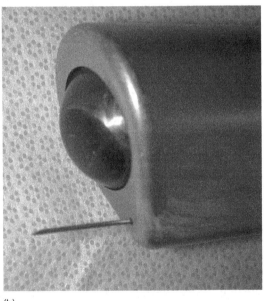

(b)

Fig. 13.9 Ovum pick-up. (a) Equipment used in OPU. (b) Detail of transducer head and needle guide. (Courtesy of Department of Animal Science and Production, University College Dublin.)

et al. (2003) found that heparin improved fertilization rates regardless of sperm separation technique in spite of observations from the bovine IVF industry which indicated that heparin may not be necessary for cryopreserved bovine sperm which have been separated through Percoll gradients.

Lechniak *et al.* (2003) reported that pre-incubation of sperm for 24 hours reduced blastocyst formation, but significantly altered the sex ratio in favour of females.

Embryo culture

Once fertilized, embryos need to be cultured to the blastocyst stage ready for non-surgical embryo transfer. Traditionally, so-called co-culture systems have been used, in which the developing embryo is grown in conjunction with cultured granulosa and/or cumulus cells. Rief *et al.* (2002) reported on the use of a novel system in which embryos were co-cultured with oviduct epithelial cells. It seems, however, that serum-containing culture systems can induce neonatal and fetal problems and there are efforts to produce synthetic, serum-free media. The problem was that cattle blastocysts developed in protein-free medium were found to be metabolically compromised (Thompson & Peterson, 2000), and various approaches have been tried to overcome this. Lane *et al.* (2003) report on the use of a serum-free physiological sequential media system which produced bovine blastocysts at rates equivalent to co-culture. Furthermore, these blastocysts had equivalent or increased cell numbers and inner cell mass development and produced equivalent pregnancy rates following transfer of both fresh and frozen IVF-produced embryos.

Problems

There are problems associated with in vitro embryo production. Low success rates limit the contribution that the procedures can make, especially to genetic improvement. Specific problems include a high incidence of polyspermy during in vitro fertilization (e.g., Mizushima & Fukui, 2001). There is also significant post-day 35 fetal loss. Thompson & Peterson (2000) found that much of this loss was due to failure of normal allantoic development within the conceptus.

Potential welfare problems related specifically to OPU have been referred to, and do not appear to be of great concern. Of much greater concern is the effect on offspring that are actually brought to term, and here there is indeed a welfare issue. Most serious is the birth of unusually large calves resulting from in vitro embryo production. Associated with this have been reports of breathing difficulties, reluctance to suckle and sudden perinatal death of calves. The reasons for this are still not clear, but the problem appears to be related to the fetus per se rather than the placenta. A number of factors have been implicated. Many of these are associated with in vitro culture procedures (e.g., Byrne *et al.*, 2002), and others include asynchronous embryo transfer and maternal exposure to high urea diets.

Reference has already been made to the possibility of altered sex ratios under certain conditions of culture during in vitro embryo production, but overall there is little evidence of significant deviation from expected ratios.

Twinning

It is normal for 1–2% of cattle pregnancies to result in the birth of twin calves. Under certain circumstances, the induction of a high proportion of twin pregnancies would offer the potential for increased reproductive efficiency. Twinning in beef cattle could improve productivity considerably. It would likewise be beneficial to obtain a high proportion of twins from dairy cows whose calves are intended to go for beef. In dairy cows that are bred to provide dairy herd replacements, twinning would only be useful if both the calves were female so that there was no possibility of freemartinism.

Three possible means of increasing the incidence of twinning are genetic selection, superovulation and embryo transfer.

Genetic selection

The incidence of twinning varies between breeds of cattle, with dairy breeds in general exhibiting a higher frequency than beef breeds. This suggests that there may be a genetic basis for the incidence of twinning. If a particular animal does have a higher than normal chance of producing twins, this chance may be enhanced by good management, and in particular by adequate nutrition. Older cows are more likely to produce twins, so that breeding and management for longevity may slightly increase the incidence of twinning in a herd. Any significant increase in twinning rates is likely to take a very long time, especially if embryo technology is not used to hasten genetic progress. Furthermore, if twinning was subsequently found to be undesirable, it would also take considerable time to breed the trait back out again. In practice, selection and management practices designed to increase the incidence of twinning are not likely to be worthwhile.

Superovulation

Twins could possibly be induced by superovulation of cows prior to insemination. As will already be apparent, the chances of controlling the superovulation rate with sufficient accuracy are slim. Immunization against the cows' own hormones may have the greatest potential as a means of inducing twinning by superovulation. Glencross *et al.* (1994), for example, showed that active immunization against inhibin resulted in increased plasma FSH concentration (presumably by suppressing the negative feedback of inhibin on pituitary FSH secretion), the development of more follicles and an increased ovulation rate as compared to control animals. However, there seems to have been little recent interest in the procedure.

Embryo transfer

The third and most likely method of producing twins in cattle is the use of embryo transfer. One approach is to transfer single embryos into a uterine horn of a cow that has been inseminated following ovulation from the contralateral ovary. The cow should thus carry her own calf plus the one resulting from the embryo transfer. This method, as with all those so far discussed, suffers from the disadvantage that the resulting calves may be of opposite sexes, which could result in freemartinism. Embryo transfer offers the possibility of avoiding this if two embryos are transferred into a non-inseminated recipient after the sex of the embryos has been determined or when the two embryos have resulted from the in vitro splitting of a fertilized embryo (see 'Cloning' below).

In general, the disadvantages of twinning (including possible freemartinism; higher risk of embryo/fetal loss; premature birth; dystocia; retained placenta; small calves) would seem to outweigh the advantages.

Cloning

Any form of asexual reproduction, either natural or by manipulation, may be defined as cloning. The offspring produced should, in theory, be genetically identical. They may not be completely so in every instance, and it is certainly possible to detect phenotypic differences between mammalian clones. For example, identical twin calves, which are naturally occurring clones, usually have different coat colour patterns at birth. Lessard *et al.* (2003) studied the semen characteristics of quadruplet bulls produced from a single egg by blastomere separation (see below). One bull showed significantly lower progressive motility and lower sperm concentration than his 'identical' brothers and the semen of another sibling froze less well than that of the other three.

Cloning could potentially be used to replicate genetically superior stock and thus help to speed the rate of genetic improvement. Careful account would need to be taken of inbreeding, of which cloning is in effect the ultimate example. However, the homogeneity resulting from cloning could lead to the creation of groups of identical cows, which could thus be fed and managed at a standard that is optimum for all of them, with positive effects on welfare as well as production. Others have considered the commercial possibilities of using cloned cattle to produce identical cuts of meat to satisfy modern supermarket demand. Cloning could also be of great value in research, considerably reducing variability due to animal differences. Furthermore, the procedure has great potential in the conservation of endangered species or breeds of animal.

Earlier cloning methods imitated the natural production of identical twins by separating the blastomeres of early developing embryos using microsurgical techniques. The zona pelucida of a two-celled embryo is incised and one of the blastomeres is removed, leaving the other to continue development within the original zona. The removed blastomere is transferred to another zona pelucida, from which an unwanted embryo has been removed. Sets of identical twins have been produced by these means. Occasionally, quadruplets can be produced by further separation of the two blastomeres of each 'twin' after its first division. Once the blastomeres from this second separation have divided, the resulting embryos will physically be two-celled, but each of the cells will be at the eight-cell stage of differentiation. Once differentiation has reached a certain point, each cell loses its ability to form a complete individual. Four is thus the theoretical limit to this technique, although in one case five identical calves were produced. Eight-cell embryos have also been divided into four pairs of cells using similar techniques with some degree of success (Willadsen & Polge, 1981).

An alternative technique of cloning individuals, with the theoretical potential to produce far more identical siblings, is to transfer nuclei from embryonic cells into enucleated oocytes. This has been possible in amphibian eggs for some years and was first achieved in mammalian (mouse) cells by McGrath & Solter in 1983. Embryos from some strains of mice yield cells (embryonic stem cells) that can be cultured over succeeding generations without differentiating. Thus, when they are transferred into recipient oocytes, they are able to contribute to the development of viable individuals. Willadsen (1986) created viable sheep embryos and demonstrated the feasibility of nuclear transfer in sheep. Single-cell eggs were bisected and the halves fused with single blastomeres from 8- and 16-cell embryos. However, the number of clones produced by this method is still restricted. It has not been possible to produce stem cell cultures, as in mice, from farm animal embryos, whose cells almost invariably differentiate as they divide. The approach in farm animals has been to inhibit or reverse the changes in chromatin structure that govern differentiation in the donor cells. Their nuclei should thus be compatible with the cytoplasm of the recipient oocyte and capable of controlling development to term.

The success of this approach was first reported by Campbell *et al.* (1996). They cultured embryonic disc cells from an ovine blastocyst and then induced quiescence by serum starvation. Recipient oocytes were prepared by arresting their development at stage II of metaphase, after which their nuclei were microsurgically removed. Donor nuclei from the embryonic disc cells were transferred into enucleated oocytes and an electric pulse used to activate the enucleated oocyte and fuse it to the donor cell. The product was embedded in agar and transferred to ligated sheep embryos for in vivo culture. Six days later, viable, dividing embryos were identified and transferred to the uteri of recipient ewes. 'Morag' and 'Megan' were cloned twins resulting from two of the embryos.

The ability to induce quiescence has enabled the production of cloned mammals from embryo, fetal and even adult cells. 'Dolly' (Wilmut *et al.*, 1997) was famous as being the first clone of an adult ewe, the donor nucleus that contributed to her genotype having come from a fibroblast from an adult sheep udder. Cloned cattle have since been produced by similar means. Currently, survival rates following nuclear transfer are less than 5%, with cumulative loss at the embryonic, fetal, perinatal and neonatal stage. Also, as with in vitro production of non-cloned embryos, abnormal offspring have been born. In spite of the reversal of differentiation in the donor, many genes may still express themselves inappropriately at different stages of development. Some improvements may be made by modifying existing techniques, but there is a need for new methods of assisting the reprogramming of transferred nuclei (Wilmut *et al.*, 2002).

Genetic engineering

Genetic engineering of lower organisms such as bacteria is now established as a commercial means of producing therapeutic and other products. For example, rennin used for milk clotting during cheese making is now biosynthesized by this means, as are many hormones used in cattle reproductive manipulation. Genetic modification has become an established, if controversial, procedure in crop production.

The basis of genetic engineering is the incorporation of an alien gene – usually from a different species – into the nucleus of a recipient. In higher mammals, if the gene is successfully incorporated into the pronucleus of a zygote it should be reproduced in every cell of the resulting conceptus and is likely to be passed on to future generations. Incorporation at any subsequent stage will result in the presence of the gene in a varying proportion of cells, creating a chimaera, which thus may not necessarily pass the gene on to its offspring.

Genetic engineering has led to the possibility of introducing new genetic material into mammalian cells, producing so-called transgenic animals. Cloning could then be used to produce further replicates of an animal shown to have successfully incorporated a desirable gene. In the livestock industry, one possible benefit would be the incorporation of genes for, say, improved production or disease resistance into groups of animals that could then be used as breeding stock for the production of further improved animals by conventional means. The protein content of milk is a characteristic that could potentially be manipulated by gene transfer, as described in the review by Wilmut *et al.* (1990). Characteristics controlled by more than one gene would be difficult to manipulate by such means. Possibly the greatest benefit from transgenic animals would be the production of therapeutic products, especially for use in human medicine, much more safely and reliably than by using transgenic bacteria or by extraction from, for example, human blood.

Wright *et al.* (1991) reported the birth of a number of transgenic sheep. One of them ('Tracy') produced viable quantities of human alpha-1-antitrypsin (AAT) in her milk, and a small flock of ewes producing substantial quantities of AAT has since been established. AAT is used in the treatment of lung disorders such as emphysema and cystic fibrosis.

The technique originally involved the injection of several hundred copies of the desired gene into the pronuclei of fertilized eggs using an extremely fine pipette. In the case of cattle, the eggs need to be centrifuged in order to see the pronuclei. Subsequently, it has been possible to improve the technique, and reduce the number of animals required, by using fetal fibroblasts as recipients of the gene. The desired gene is transferred along with a marker gene, such as one that imparts resistance to specific bacteria, to evaluate incorporation. The transgenic cells are used as donors for nuclear transfer to enucleated oocytes.

This modification was used in a further breakthough reported by Schnieke *et al.* (1997) who produced a live sheep ('Polly'), which was a clone of a fibroblast that had successfully incorporated the gene for production of human factor IX.

A huge amount of investigation needs to be carried out before cloning and genetic engineering can be carried out reliably and repeatedly. As with most technology, there will be debate as to whether the advantages outweigh the costs and drawbacks. These techniques more than most are also subject to a great deal of ethical debate. On balance, it is likely that the technologies will make a significant contribution to livestock production and welfare at some time in the future.

References

Båge, R., Petyim, S., Larsson, B., Hallap, T., Bergqvist, A.S., Gustafsson, H. & Rodríguez-Martínez, H. (2003) *Reproduction Fertility and Development*, **15**, 115–123.

Boland, M.P., Lonergan, P. & Sreenan, J.M. (2000) In *Fertility in the High-Producing Dairy Cow* (ed. M.G. Diskin). *British Society of Animal Science Occasional Publication*, **26**, 263–275.

Brackett, B.G., Bousquet, D., Boice, M.L., Donawick, W.J., Evans, J.E. & Dressel, M.A. (1982) *Biology of Reproduction*, **27**, 147.

Bredbacka, P.J., Kankaanpaa, A. & Peippo, J. (1995) *Theriogenology*, **44**, 167–176.

Byrne, A.T., Southgate, J., Brison, D.R. & Leese, H.J. (2002) *Molecular Reproduction and Development*, **62**, 489–495.

Campbell, K.H.S., McWhir, J., Ritchie, W.A. & Wilmut, I. (1996) *Nature*, **380**, 64–66.

Chastant-Maillard, S., Quinton, H., Lauffenburger, J., Cordonnier-Lefort, N., Richard, C., Marchal, J., Mormede, P. & Renard, J.P. (2003) *Reproduction*, **125**, 555–563.

Claycomb, R.W., Delwiche, M.J., Munro, C.J. & BonDurant, R.H. (1995) *American Society of Agricultural Engineers Paper No. **95-3564***, St Joseph, USA.

Gillis, E.H., Sreenan, J.M. & Kane, M. (2002) *Proceedings of the Sixth International Conference on Domestic Ruminants*, Crieff Hydro, August, A26.

Glencross, R.G., Bleach, E.C., Wood, S.C. & Knight, P.G. (1994) *Journal of Reproduction and Fertility*, **100**, 599–605.

Goodhand, K.L., Watt, R.G., Staines, M.E., Hutchinson, J.S.M. & Broadbent, P.J. (1999) *Theriogenology*, **51**, 951–961.

Gordon, I. (1994) *Laboratory Production of Cattle Embryos*. CAB International, University Press, Cambridge.

Heape, W. (1890) *Proceedings of the Royal Society*, **28**, 457.

Howes, E.A., Miller, N.G., Dolby, C., Hutchings, A., Butcher, G.W. & Jones, R. (1997) *Journal of Reproduction and Fertility*, **110**, 195–204.

Kiddy, C.A., Mitchell, D.S., Bolt, D.J. & Hawk, H.W. (1978) *Biology of Reproduction*, **19**, 389.

Koelsch, R.K., Aneshansley, D.J. & Butler, W.R. (1994) *Journal of Agricultural Engineering Research*, **58**, 115–120.

Lane, M., Gardner, D.K., Hasler, M.J. & Hasler, J.F. (2003) *Theriogenology*, **60**, 407–419.

Lechniak, D., Strabel, T., Bousquet, D. & King, A.W. (2003) *Reproduction in Domestic Animals*, **38**, 224–227.

Lessard, C., Masseau, I., Bilodeau, J.F., Kroetsch, T., Twagiramungu, H., Bailey, J.L., Leclerc, P. & Sullivan, R. (2003) *Theriogenology*, **59**, 1865–1877.

McEvoy, T.G. & Sinclair, K.D. (1997) *Scottish Agricultural College Animal Science Research Report*.

McEvoy, T.G., Gebbie, F.E., Sinclair, K.D., Dolman, D.F., Thain, A.W., Watt, R.G., Higgins, L.C. & Broadbent, P.J. (1996) *Journal of Reproduction and Fertility Abstract Series*, **18**, 32.

McEvoy, T.G., Thompson, H., Dolman, D.F., Watt, R.G., Reis, A. & Staines, M.E. (2002) *Veterinary Record*, **151**, 653–658.

McGrath, J. & Solter, D. (1983) *Science*, **220**, 1300–1302.

Mendes, J.O., Burns, P.D., De La Torre-Sanchez, J.F. & Seidel, G.E. (2003) *Theriogenology*, **60**, 331–340.

Merton, J.S., de Roos, A.P.W., Mullaart, E., de Ruigh, L., Kaal, L., Vos, P.L.A.M. & Dieleman, S.J. (2003) *Theriogenology*, **59**, 651–674.

Mizushima, S. & Fukui, Y. (2001) *Theriogenology*, **55**, 1431–1445.

Mottram, T.T., Lark, R.M., Wathes, D.C., Persaud, K.C., Swan, M. & Cooper, J.M. (2000) In *Proceedings of International Symposium on Electronic Noses and Olfaction* (eds J.W. Gardner & K.C. Persaud), Brighton, UK, July.

Mutter, L.R., Graden, A.P. & Olds, D. (1964) *Artificial Insemination Digest*, **12**, 3.

Pemberton, R.M, Hart, J.P. & Mottram, T.T. (2001) *Biosensors and Bioelectronics*, **16**, 715–723.

Pieterse, M.C., Vos, P.L.A.M., Kruip, T.A.M., Wurth, Y.A., Van Beneden, T.H, Willemse, A.H. & Taverne, M.A.M. (1991) *Theriogenology*, **35**, 19–24.

Rief, S., Sinowatz, F., Stojkovic, M., Einspanier, R., Wolf, E. & Prelle, K. (2002) *Reproduction*, **124**, 543–556.

Rieger, D. (1984) *Theriogenology*, **21**, 138–149.

Roth, Z., Arav, A., Braw-tal, R., Bor, A. & Wolfenson, D. (2002) *Journal of Dairy Science*, **85**, 1398–1405.

Rowson, L.E.A., Moore, R.M. & Lawson, R.A.S. (1969) *Journal of Reproduction and Fertility*, **18**, 517.

Schnieke, A.E., Kind, A.J., Ritchie, W.A., Mycock, K., Scott, A.R., Ritchie, M., Wilmut, I., Colman, A. & Campbell, K.H. (1997) *Science*, **278**, 2130–2133.

Seidel, G.E. (2002) *Reproduction*, **124**, 533–743.

Seidel, G.E. (2003) *Theriogenology*, **59**, 585–598.

Shea, B.F. (1999) *Theriogenology*, **51**, 841–854.

Sreenan, J.M. (1983) *Veterinary Record*, **112**, 494.

Thompson, J.G. & Peterson, A.J. (2000) *Human Reproduction*, **15** (Suppl. 5), 59–67.

Utsumi, K. & Iritani, A. (1993) *Molecular Reproduction and Development*, **36**, 238–241.

Vajta, G., Holm, P., Kuwayama, M., Booth, P.J., Jacobsen, H., Greve, T. & Callesen, H. (1998) *Molecular Reproduction and Development*, **51**, 53–58.

White, K.L. & Anderson, G.B. (1987) *Biology of Reproduction*, **37**, 867–873.

Willadsen, S.M. (1986) *Nature*, **320**, 63–65.

Willadsen, S.M. & Polge, C. (1981) *Veterinary Record*, **108**, 211–213.

Willett, E.L., Black, W.O., Casida, L.E., Stone, W.H. & Buckner, P.J. (1951) *Science*, **113**, 247.

Williams, T.J. (1986) *Theriogenology*, **25**, 733–739.

Wilmut, I., Archibald, A.L., Harris, S., McClenaghan, M., Simons, J.P., Whitelaw, C.B.A. & Clark, A.J. (1990) *Theriogenology*, **33**, 113–121.

Wilmut, I., Schnieke, A.E., McWhir, J., Kind, A.J. & Campbell, H.S. (1997) *Nature*, **385**, 810–812.

Wilmut, I., de Sousa, P., Dinnyes, A., King, T.J., Paterson, L.A., Singh, P.B., Wells, D.N. & Young, L.E. (2002) *Nature*, **419**, 583–586.

Winterberger-Torres, S. & Popescu, C. (1980) *Theriogenology*, **14**, 309–318.

Wright, G., Carver, A., Cottom, D., Reeves, D., Scott, A., Simons, P., Wilmut, I., Garner, I. & Colman, A. (1991) *Biotechnology*, **9**, 830–834.

Chapter 14
Reproductive Management

In order to maximize efficiency, and specifically reproductive efficiency, in a dairy or beef herd the farmer should (1) develop a series of targets, (2) manage the herd and individual cows so as to best achieve those targets efficiently and (3) evaluate performance on a regular, ongoing basis, in order to correct problems before they have too serious an impact on the attainment of the targets.

The targets that need to be aimed for fall into a number of overall categories:

- culling and replacement policy
- the rearing of heifer replacements
- calving patterns.

Culling and replacement policy

The dairy herd

Even if a dairy herd is not increasing in size, it is still necessary to bring new animals into the herd every year to replace those that are culled. The policy for culling cows from the herd can have dramatic effects on the reproductive performance of the herd. Culling may be planned, i.e., deliberate policy, or unplanned, e.g., following disease or injury.

To maximize genetic progress, a high proportion of cows should be culled each year and replaced with (hopefully!) higher genetic merit heifers. A rigorous culling policy may also be appropriate in some circumstances, particularly to tighten a block or seasonal calving pattern. For example, this can be an effective method of achieving and maintaining a compact calving period in the beef herd. On the other hand, cows need to remain in the herd for five or more lactations to maximize economic returns, and heifers in their first, second and even third lactations will not be yielding up to their genetic potential. Thus, culling rates should never exceed 25%, and we suggest 20%, equivalent to five lactations per cow, as a better aim. Culling rates greater than 20% are not advisable in dairy herds since:

- There would be a higher proportion of first-calved heifers in the herds, therefore reducing average milk yield.
- The higher the culling rate, the more heifers have to be reared, thus requiring more resources.

Table 14.1 Reasons for culling.

Country	Percentage of total culls due to			
	Fertility	Mastitis	Lameness	Yield
UK[a]	25.3	16.3	7.7	9.0
UK[b]	36.5[e]	10.1	5.6	11.5
France[c]	28.4	12.4	2.7	16.7
Canada[d]: Holsteins	27–29	14–17	—	—
Canada[d]: Ayrshires	23–25	14–17	—	—

[a] Whitaker *et al.* (2000)
[b] Esslemont and Kossaibati (1997).
[c] Seegers *et al.* (1998)
[d] Van Doormal & Brand (2003).
[e] Large herds: 8.7% of all cows culled each year due to fertility problems.

It is clearly desirable to reduce the level of unplanned culling so that planned culling of poor yielders or temperamental cows can be carried out. Unfortunately the average herd life in the UK is now no more than 2.5 lactations and much less in the USA. If the herd's fertility status is good it should only be necessary to replace 5% of the cows each year due to reproductive problems and cows should mainly be culled for relatively low yield and/or old age. Esslemont *et al.* (2000) reported that 14% of cows in the UK were culled owing to reproductive problems and in many countries fertility is easily the most common reason for culling. Failure to conceive and other problems, especially associated with feet and udders, lead to a large number of 'involuntary culls', so that there is often little or no choice of cows to cull in order to select for improvement (see Table 14.1). The UK figures for the proportion of culls due to fertility problems contrast badly with the figure of 19% quoted in our second edition (MMB, 1984).

Cows culled for 'infertility' are usually described as barren. However, the majority of cows culled for infertility reasons are likely to be perfectly normal anatomically and capable of becoming pregnant given the right management.

Replacements may be bought in as in-calf or newly calved heifers or cows. The potential of such animals could be more uncertain than that of home-produced stock. Also, the new animals could either introduce disease into the herd or fall victim to a disease that is endemic in the cows already in the herd and to which they are immune. For these and other considerations, especially economic ones, replacements are often reared from calves born within the herd. Mainly as a precaution against disease, some herds aim to remain completely 'closed', rearing all replacements from within the herd and never buying in stock from outside the herd.

Choice of calves for rearing

An ideal herd of, say, 100 cows should produce 100 calves each year, approximately half of them being female. Thus, for a 25% replacement rate, only half of the heifer calves born each year would be needed for rearing. It would thus be possible to choose the best calves, as judged by their appearance, the performance and pedigree of the dam and the bull with which she was inseminated. More on this aspect will be found in Chapter 15 on selection of animals for breeding. If cows are very high yielding, and are allowed longer lactations, fewer calves will be produced per year on average, but the need for replacements would be reduced in proportion.

In practice it is often necessary to rear nearly all the available heifer calves. The choice may be even more restricted if only calves born in certain months of the year are suitable for rearing, as will be discussed shortly.

The rearing of replacement heifers

Targets for rearing

Up to a point, the two main requirements in rearing replacement heifers are (1) that they should grow at a rapid rate and (2) that they should calve at as early an age as possible. The former obviously influences the latter to a certain extent.

Rapid growth

The replacement heifer needs to grow so that she becomes able to reproduce efficiently and to produce reasonable quantities of milk. Just before first calving, Friesian heifers should weigh around 510 kg. This necessitates an average liveweight gain of 0.64 kg/day from the time of birth. The rate of gain should be less during the first 5–6 months of life (around 0.5 kg) to avoid subsequent depression of milk yields. Slower growth during the winter months is also acceptable, since compensatory growth can occur on the cheaper feed provided by grazing the following spring.

Early age at first calving

The earlier that heifers calve, the sooner they can replace cull cows in the milking herd and the quicker will be the rate of genetic gain in the herd (assuming the replacements are superior to the culls). Today the target age at first calving is approximately two years.

The earlier replacements calve, the fewer there will be on the farm at any one time. In a 100-cow herd with a 25% replacement rate, for example, there will be around 75 replacements due to calve at three years of age, but only 50 if they will be calving at two years. Consequently, if replacement heifers calve at an earlier age they will overall be less of a drain on the farm's resources, so that they could be used to support more milking cows or other enterprises. It is true to say that, within limits, the earlier in life that heifers start to produce milk, the higher will be their lifetime production. Finally, it seems that if heifers are too old at first calving, they may be more likely to suffer dystocia, perhaps because of excessive weight gain.

Calves born after December in autumn-calving herds and after February in spring-calving herds will not reach 23 months of age by the required month of calving and will thus need to calve at nearer three years of age if they are to fit the herd's calving pattern. This can add considerably to rearing costs. In addition, a calf born later than February will not be able to take advantage of summer grazing during its first year.

Thus it can be seen that the provision of calves to rear for replacements in seasonally calving herds depends initially on the reproductive efficiency of the milking herd. Physiological, environmental and managemental factors affecting reproduction must be optimized to provide calves suitable for rearing at the right time of year. The pressure is reduced if two herds under the same management, or two groups in the same herd, calve in two different seasons. First-calf heifers would enter the herd or group most suited to their calving date. The problem is obviously minimized in herds with no marked seasonal calving pattern.

Insemination of replacement heifers

Ideally a heifer should be gaining weight at a rate of slightly above average around the time of service. Friesian heifers, which are able to calve at around two years, should weigh approximately 330 kg and be increasing in weight by about 0.7 kg/day. Underweight heifers are more likely to conceive if they are on a high plane of nutrition and increasing in weight, whilst those that are overweight should be stable or losing weight.

Oestrus detection can be a bigger problem in heifers than in cows, partly because they are handled and observed less frequently. Two possible ways of addressing this are (1) the use of a bull and (2) synchronization of oestrus.

The use of a bull

The herdsperson may not wish to use expensive semen in a heifer until she has started to lactate and given a tangible guide to her potential. Thus one of the main advantages of AI (maximum genetic gain), discussed in Chapter 15, may not apply. However, the other drawbacks associated with the use of a bull must be taken into account.

Synchronization of oestrus

It has been shown that heifers are more likely than lactating cows to respond normally to luteolysing treatments using prostaglandin or prostaglandin analogues (see Chapter 9). This means that oestrus synchronization based on such luteolysis is not only more desirable but also likely to be more effective in heifers than in cows.

Oestrus detection is often more difficult in heifers than in cows because management techniques decrease the chances of observing a heifer in oestrus, and also because the heifers in themselves can cause problems. For example, it has been found in practice that indiscriminate mounting in a group of heifers can remove tail paste from most of the heifers whether or not they are in heat. It may therefore be appropriate to treat heifers with two injections of prostaglandin 10–12 days apart and inseminate them all three and four days after the second injection (the 'two plus two' method is described in Chapter 9).

An approach that has been used successfully at the SAC, for example, is to synchronize groups of heifers (in this case with a progesterone ear implant) and then, about 32 days after insemination, pregnancy diagnosis is carried out by ultrasound scan. Any heifers found not pregnant should be in mid-cycle and can be resynchronized with a single prostaglandin injection followed by fixed-time insemination.

The need for oestrus detection is obviated with synchronization, but there are dangers. If, for example, a stress factor such as a severe thunderstorm should occur at the time of service, the chance of conception could be reduced for the entire group of heifers. Another danger in a large group of heifers is that the inseminator may become fatigued, and thus less efficient as his or her work proceeds. Finally, assuming conception rates are satisfactory and the heifers calve over a short space of time, there is a further danger of putting too much pressure on resources needed at calving. Natural variation in gestation lengths may be sufficient to overcome this.

Whether or not oestrus is synchronized it is important to avoid undue stress when inseminating both heifers and lactating cows. If heifers are not used to being handled, the trauma can be greater and the consequences for conception even more severe. Heifers should be accustomed to handling and premises should be designed for efficient movement and restraint of animals for AI. Operations should also be planned to avoid undue noise and excitement at and around the critical time of insemination.

Introduction to the herd

The combination of being introduced to an unfamiliar group of older and more dominant females, producing a calf, the onset of lactation and being milked in a strange environment can cause severe physiological and psychological stress to a heifer. Everything possible should be done to minimize this trauma. It is good practice to introduce the heifer to the herd about two weeks before calving to acquaint her with the new environment. It is also important to adjust feeding so as to avoid a sudden change at the onset of lactation. As with all cows, the newly calved heifer needs to be well fed to enable high milk yield and to support another pregnancy within two to three months. The first-calf heifer also needs feed for further growth, especially if she has calved at two years of age. Adequate nutrition is therefore essential, but again it must be stressed that this should not be achieved by a sudden change on or around the day of calving.

Stress around the time of calving lowers the animal's resistance to disease. The need for feeding properly to avoid metabolic disease is implicit in the previous paragraphs and the subject is covered more fully in veterinary and nutritional textbooks. Apart from this, the calving heifer is also more susceptible to infectious disease, particularly of the uterus and mammary gland. A clean and comfortable calving box is an important aid in the prevention of infection in both the calf and the cow unless she calves outside.

Recent findings suggest that heifers being reared should have sufficient contact with the main herd to be able to contract and build up resistance to infections endemic in the lactating animals. In order to minimize stress during the critical first lactation, the possibility of handling them as a separate group should be considered.

Beef heifers

The majority of the above points relate to beef heifers as well as to dairy heifers; however, there are one or two additional specific points relating to beef heifers.

Since in the UK the majority of suckler cows are of crossbred beef on dairy type, e.g., Hereford × Friesian, most suckler herd replacement heifers originate from the dairy herd. Most commercial suckler producers buy replacements as bulling heifers or as down-calvers. Rearing dairy-bred heifers is probably the most economic method of providing replacements, but it may not be practicable particularly if only small numbers are required.

As discussed above, the date of first calving is important in determining the future calving patterns of the herd. It is usual practice to ensure that first-calving heifers calve 2–3 weeks before the rest of the herd.

The use of heavy breeds of bull, such as Charolais, Simmental and South Devon, on maiden heifers should be avoided due to potential problems of dystocia (see Chapter 12).

Calving patterns

The dairy herd

The dairy farmer has three main options when deciding on a suitable calving pattern:

- Block calving. Cows are bred to calve over a very short period of time.
- Seasonal calving. Cows are bred so that they only calve in a particular season of the year.
- All-year-round calving.

These options are described and discussed in Chapter 1.

There is also an element of choice in the intended calving interval. For many cows, the aim should still be 365 days. It may be difficult or undesirable to aim for such a short interval in some very high yielding cows. If intervals are longer, block or seasonal calving patterns are less appropriate. Some managers overcome this by calving in two or more blocks, with long calving interval cows being allowed to 'slip back' into later calving blocks.

The beef suckler herd

Beef cow herds are often managed to calve on a seasonal basis. In the UK, for example, herds traditionally calve in either spring or autumn. Autumn-calving herds tend to produce a higher gross margin per cow than spring-calving herds under UK conditions, due mainly to a greater output. However, spring-calving herds tend to be stocked more heavily and thus there is little difference in gross margins expressed on a per hectare basis.

The calf is virtually the sole product of the beef herd and therefore the rate of calf production is even more critical than it is in the dairy herd. A 365-day calving interval is optimal, but a compact calving season is also desirable, as is discussed in Chapter 1.

Management to achieve reproductive targets

As a basic rule of thumb, cows should be served as soon as possible after day 60 postpartum. If the oestrus detection rate is approximately 75% and there are no disease problems, then an average 365-day interval should be achieved with little variation (see Chapter 1). There is often a temptation to start inseminating earlier, in case a subsequent oestrus is not detected. Fig. 12.9 illustrates the dangers of this. Conception rates are likely to be lower, and subsequent death of the conceptus will be more likely, especially in high-yielding cows. In herds served too soon, the result may be that the average calving interval is close to 365 but that the variation is rather large. In other words, there will be cows with calving intervals both well below and well in excess of 365 days.

If the calving to conception interval is much less than 85 days (i.e., a 365-day calving interval), the presence of the fetus has a tendency to depress milk yield when it should be near maximum and at the end of lactation the cow will have to be dried off sooner than normal, while milk production is still high. It is also likely that the dry period would be too short to allow proper regeneration of the udder so that production will be low in the ensuing lactation.

Conception later than 85 days after calving will lead to calving intervals greater than 365 days, with serious economic consequences for many cows. However, Taylor *et al.* (2003) showed that high-yielding cows could continue to lose body condition until at least 100 days after calving. Coffey *et al.* (2002) found that energy balance, calculated from daily measures of feed intake and milk output, returned to positive values at days 72, 75 and 95 in lactations 1, 2 and 3, respectively. It is thus clear that some cows not only achieve good economic performance at calving intervals of more than 365 days, but also will have difficulty conceiving and maintaining their pregnancy if they are served on or before 85 days postpartum. In year-round-calving herds, choosing individual calving to intended start of service intervals should be considered. Cows of moderate genetic index with low or average yield expectations should be served as soon as possible after 60 days postpartum if they are healthy and in good body condition. A number of factors individually or combined could suggest an extension of this voluntary waiting period. They include:

- high percentage of Holstein blood
- predicted yields of 9000 litres or more
- very high genetic index
- higher lactation number – especially fourth or greater
- dystocia or retained placenta.

Further delays should be considered if the cow is ill, lame or in very low condition score at the originally planned date.

Breeding policy

There are three main choices for inseminating cows:

(1) *Allow a fertile bull to run with the herd all year round.* This is the simplest fertility management system, and its main advantages are:
- The detection and recording of oestrus are not necessary.
- No decisions on the timing of insemination are required.
- No manpower or facilities are needed to restrain animals for AI.

However, this method has a number of disadvantages:

- The herd does not have access to bulls of exceptional genetic merit.
- There is a high risk of venereally transmitted diseases (see Chapter 12).
- It is possible that the cows may be served at the wrong time, e.g., too early postpartum, leading to excessively short, uneconomic calving intervals.
- The time of expected calving may not be known, which makes management planning very difficult.
- Cows with reproductive problems, e.g., repeat breeders, and those with cystic ovaries may remain undetected for long periods.
- If the bull is subfertile there could be a long delay before this is detected, resulting in serious consequences for the reproductive performance of the herd.

(2) *Hand mating.* A bull is used to inseminate individually selected cows when they are due for service. This system also entails the risk of spreading venereal diseases and the cost of rearing and maintaining a dangerous and otherwise non-productive animal that is unlikely to aid good genetic progress in the herd. In addition, it can be very labour intensive, but it does at least overcome the last four disadvantages above.

(3) *Artificial insemination.* This has a number of clear advantages over natural service, including:
   - Genetic gain.
   - Cost effectiveness – a bull is expensive to rear, house and maintain.
   - Disease control, the main reason for the original introduction of AI.
   - Safety.
   - Flexibility. Different bulls can be chosen to meet different needs.
   - Fertility control. The time of service can be controlled and recorded, enabling future procedures, such as drying off, to be planned accordingly. As with hand mating, there is scope for decision on calving patterns.

As discussed in Chapter 10, there is a further choice to be made between AI by technician service and 'do it yourself' AI, or possibly a combination of both.

In herds that practise AI and also maintain a bull, he can be used as a 'sweeper' to run with cows that are known not to be pregnant after a number of services or run with the herd after a certain date to serve any cows that are not already pregnant. Remember that he should also be housed where he can be of use to aid oestrus detection.

Disease control

We have shown (Chapter 12) that infectious diseases, such as campylobacteriosis (vibriosis), infectious bovine rhinotracheitis (IBR) and bovine virus diarrhoea (BVD), can seriously affect reproduction. Good hygiene and management should always be practised to minimize the risk of introducing infection and the appropriate vaccination procedures should be vigorously followed. If a cow is ill, this should be rectified before attempting to inseminate her.

It is clearly essential to remedy any infectious problem before attempting to improve herd reproductive performance by other means.

Nutritional management

Nutritional status is of vital importance in the maintenance of a high rate of reproductive performance. The nutrition of cattle is covered more comprehensively in specialized texts and only the basic principles will be described here.

The fundamental requirements for optimum fertility are that negative energy balance is minimized, as is excessive deposition and mobilization of body fat. The technique of body condition scoring has been developed as a simple, semisubjective monitor of cows' body reserves. Cows are scored by manual palpation of the quantity of subcutaneous fat cover on various parts of the body. Methods were developed about 25 years ago for both dairy [National Institute for Research into Dairying (NIRD): ADAS, 1978; DEFRA, 2001] and beef cows (Lowman *et al.*, 1976) and although the finer details vary slightly, the overall principle is the same. The thickness of fat cover over the tailhead and lumbar area (see Fig. 14.1) is estimated and assigned a score from 0 (emaciated) to 5 (very fat). A practical guide to condition scoring, based on the NIRD system and used in ADAS and Semex courses, is shown in Table 14.2.

Cows should be fed to calve at a condition score of 2.5–3.5 and should then lose minimum condition until conception (see Table 14.3). Calving cows in fatter condition may cause difficulties which may lead to delayed involution, reproductive tract damage, susceptibility to infection of the tract or a combination of these problems. Also, cows with a score of 4 or more are likely to mobilize their fat reserves excessively during the early postpartum period. In dairy cows this situation can lead to metabolic problems, particularly the excessive accumulation of fat in the liver (the 'fatty liver' syndrome) and to problems with subsequent conception. On the other hand, cows calving with a low condition score are likely to be severely deficient in energy by the time of intended conception, as it is then very difficult for them to eat enough feed for the demands of lactation. Both dairy and beef cows calving at a low body condition score undergo prolonged periods before the onset of ovarian cyclicity (see Chapter 12). Consequently, conception is likely to be seriously delayed in such cows.

If the calving score is correct, it will be more easy to achieve the target score at service (2+), which is the most critical, as it is most closely related to reproductive performance (see Table 14.3). It has been shown that the calving

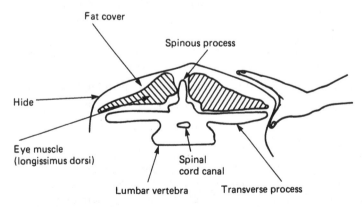

Fig. 14.1 The technique of body condition scoring of cattle over the lumbar vertebrae.

Table 14.2 Dairy cow condition scoring. Score the tailhead first. If the loin score is the same, or only half a score different, use the tailhead score without adjustment. If the loin score is at least one point different, adjust the tailhead score by half a point to obtain the final score. The final score is never more than half a point different from the tailhead score. Score regularly, and not just by eye, which can be misleading.

Score	Tailhead	Loin
0	Deep cavity; skin tightly stretched over bones	No fatty tissue; transverse process (TP) shapes clear; emaciated
1	Deep depression on either side of tailhead; no fatty tissue; skin supple	TP ends sharp; upper surfaces felt easily; deep depression
2	Shallow cavity lined with fatty tissue; pelvis felt easily	TP ends rounded; upper surfaces felt with pressure; depression
3	Fatty tissue easily felt over whole area; skin smooth; pelvis can be felt	TP ends felt with pressure; thick tissue on upper surface; slight depression
4	Folds of soft fatty tissue; patches of fat under skin; pelvis felt with pressure	TP ends cannot be felt; no depression
5	Tailhead buried in fatty tissue; skin distended; pelvis cannot be felt	Folds of fatty tissue over TPs; bones cannot be felt

Table 14.3 Recommended target body condition scores of cows at various stages of the reproductive cycle.

	Mating	Mid-pregnancy	Calving
Autumn-calving suckler cows[a]	2.5	2	3
Spring-calving suckler cows[a]	2.5	3	2.5
Dairy cows[b]	2+	3–3.5	3–3.5

[a] MLC (1981).
[b] ADAS (1978).

interval is negatively correlated with body condition at the time of mating in beef cows (see Fig. 14.2) although the true relationship is probably curvilinear. This target score is also most difficult to achieve in autumn-calving cows as they are mated during mid-winter when they are lactating and when good quality feed is expensive. In contrast, the nutritional drain of lactation is offset in spring-calvers by the plentiful supply of grazing.

A high-yielding dairy cow in early lactation is very likely to be in a 'negative energy balance', so that body reserves are being utilized. The chances of conception are improved when the peak of lactation is passed and the cow's current energy intake is greater than the output. These short-term changes cannot be detected by condition scoring. This situation again supports the argument for not attempting to serve cows too early after parturition.

As pregnancy progresses the lactational demand for a high level of feed decreases. This enables the cow to replace body energy reserves that were lost during early lactation. Thus the cow can be brought back towards the target body condition score for the subsequent calving. As parturition approaches, the

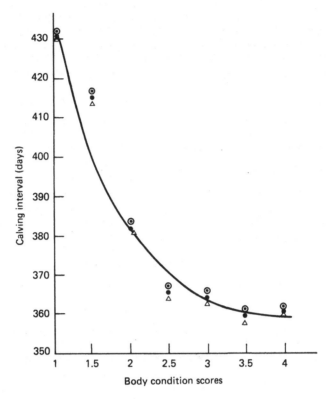

Fig. 14.2 Relationship between body condition score at mating and calving interval in beef cows. Circles containing dots indicate beef × Friesian cows; solid circles indicate mean; triangles indicate beef cows.

feed level should be adjusted so that weight gain is not excessive in order to avoid the problems of over-fat cows referred to above.

Stress

The nature of stress and its effects on reproduction were discussed in Chapter 12. Broadly speaking, factors that compromise welfare increase stress and decrease the chances of achieving reproductive targets. Causes of stress include lameness and other illnesses, sudden changes in nutrition, mishandling or sudden fright and a variety of other factors. Stress can affect reproduction at almost any stage from calving until the next pregnancy is well established (approximately two months post-conception). Critical areas include:

- around the time of ovulation: reduced oestrus intensity; interference with ovulation
- the first few days after fertilization: impaired progesterone production

- the first two months of pregnancy (especially about 30–50 days after conception), when embryo and early fetal loss can occur
- calving.

Care should be taken to avoid any upset to cows at these times. Careful handling of cows at AI includes the need for well-designed facilities. Sudden changes of nutrition should be avoided at critical times. Cows should not, for example, be switched into different feed groups at critical times, when psychological, physical and nutritional factors associated with changes in social structure may upset conception or pregnancy.

Provided that other nutritional and managemental factors are adequate, cows that are used to a quiet and constant routine at all times are likely to have the least problems with reproduction.

Hormonal manipulation

Induction of ovarian cycles

A delay in the onset of ovarian cycles can lead to extended calving intervals and possible increased variation between cows within a herd. A reliable method of induction of ovulation in acyclic cows could be of advantage in allowing the early rebreeding of late calving cows (see Chapter 12). However, no consistently successful treatments have yet been developed, and in any case it is better, where possible, to allow the cow to return naturally to cyclicity once the effects of early lactation negative energy balance and stress have been overcome.

Synchronization of oestrus

A number of procedures have been developed for the synchronization of oestrus (see Chapter 9 and discussion of the pros and cons). Generally speaking, synchronization is more appropriate in dairy heifers and in beef heifers and cows and, fortuitously, these animals respond best to synchronization. We consider it more appropriate to inseminate lactating dairy cows at a naturally occurring ovulation, following the detection of oestrus (or, possibly, ovulation as determined by progesterone levels). Hormonal treatments can be used judiciously to correct specific problems in individual cows.

Veterinary intervention

Good health in the herd is vital to good reproductive performance and the veterinary surgeon should play a key role in both prevention and cure of disease. Whether regular veterinary visits (as opposed to call-out on demand for treatments, PDs, etc.) are advisable is a matter of individual circumstance. Economic assessments of their value have given conflicting results.

Advantages include:

- PDs will be kept up to date
- identification and examination of potential problem cows
- veterinary involvement in reproductive management
- good management of cows and expenses.

Disadvantages include:

- urgent treatments may be delayed until routine visit
- expense
- timing of PDs, etc.

Oestrus detection

Where AI is used, the detection of oestrus at the appropriate time of the ovarian cycle is vital. Failure to detect oestrus is a major cause of poor reproductive performance and this has already been discussed in detail in Chapter 8.

Recording of reproductive performance

The keeping of accurate records is necessary for good herd reproductive management. Recording systems have been developed to a more sophisticated state for dairy cows, but records are equally important to maximize fertility in the beef herd. A number of types of recording systems are available. They include:

- a simple diary
- event recording sheet
- display board
- computer systems
- individual cow cards.

The type of system used is not important as long as it is straightforward and convenient to use. The information that should be recorded (input) should include at a minimum:

- cow identity
- calving date
- oestrus (bulling) dates
- earliest date for service
- service date
- bull used for service
- result of pregnancy diagnosis
- other veterinary treatments.

The recording system should be capable of quickly providing the following information (output):

- cows ready for service
- cows not served by target date
- cows ready for pregnancy diagnosis
- cows pregnant
- cows to be dried off (dairy)
- cows due to calve.

Whilst a number of commercial computer recording and analysis packages are now available, the simple recording of information on the farm is still necessary. In addition to the output data described above these commercial packages usually provide periodic summaries of herd fertility status.

In summary, records are important since they enable the farmer (1) to monitor the reproductive performance of the herd and of the individual cows and (2) to take action on the basis indicated by the records. Two particular and important uses of records are (1) the recording of all oestrus events, including supplementary signs such as bleeding, to predict approximate dates of expected oestrus and highlight problem cows and (2) the recording of all problems as an aid to culling decisions.

Evaluation of success

It is extremely important to estimate the efficiency of reproduction in both the dairy and the beef herd. Many farmers do not know how well their cows are reproducing. They may therefore be losing considerable sums of money, and are not in a position to take appropriate remedial action. A number of parameters have traditionally been used to evaluate reproductive performance. These include:

- *Calving interval.* An average calving interval is a poor means of assessing success. It may include intervals that are uneconomically short as well as those that are too long. Furthermore, it takes no account of cows that should have become pregnant, but failed to do so.
- *Conception rates.* These fail to take account of cows that were not served, or that had unacceptably long delays to service, as a result of poor oestrus detection.
- *Pregnancy rates.* This is a slightly better measure, since it calculates the percentage of cows intended for service that actually become pregnant, but still does not reflect the detrimental effect of overlong calving intervals caused by poor heat detection and conception rates.
- *Culling rates.* These again do not reflect abnormally long calving intervals.

Reproductive efficiency (fertility factor) is a useful parameter since it compares performance with target. It includes all cows that are intended to become pregnant and takes account of different objectives, such as deliberately long intervals for very high-yielding cows. The figure is arrived at as follows:

- Calculate submission rate – the percentage of cows that are inseminated within 23 days of the day they were due for service. The aim is 80%.
- Calculate pregnancy rate – the percentage of inseminations that result in a positive pregnancy diagnosis. Seventy per cent should still be a realistic aim, in spite of rates currently being achieved.
- Multiply the two to get reproductive efficiency. This should be at least 50%.

Cu-sums, which graph success rates over time, are useful for keeping track of submission and conception rates on a continuing basis, and can help to highlight developing problems in time for remedial action to be taken.

References

ADAS (1978) *Advisory Leaflet*, No. 612.
Coffey, M.P., Simm, G. & Brotherstone, S. (2002) *Journal of Dairy Science*, **85**, 2669–2678.
DEFRA (2001) *Condition Scoring of Dairy Cows*.
Esslemont, R.J. & Kossaibati, M.A. (1997) *Veterinary Record*, **140**, 36–39.
Esslemont, R.J., Kossaibati, M.A. & Allcock, J. (2000) *British Society of Animal Science Occasional Publication*, **26**, 19–29.
Kilkenny, J.B. (1979) *World Review of Animal Production*, **14**, 65.
Lowman, B.G., Scott, N.A. & Somerville, S.M. (1976) *East of Scotland College of Agriculture Bulletin*, **6**.
MLC (1981) *Beef Production Yearbook*.
MMB (1984) *Report of the Breeding and Production Organisation* 1983/84.
Seegers, H., Beaudeau, F., Fourichon, C. & Bareille, N. (1998) *Preventative Veterinary Medicine*, **36**, 257–271.
Taylor, V.J., Beever, D.E., Bryant, M.J. & Wathes, D.C. (2003) *Theriogenology*, **59**, 1661–1677.
Van Doormal, B. & Brand, P. (2003) *Canadian Dairy Network*.
Whitaker, D.A., Kelly, J.M. & Smith, S. (2000) *Veterinary Record*, **146**, 363–367.

Chapter 15
Selection for Breeding

The choice or selection of parents to create future generations is obviously of crucial importance in determining the future productivity of the herd and may also have an impact on future reproductive performance. This chapter therefore discusses briefly how selection decisions may be made.

Individual bulls can be used to sire a large number of calves. A bull used in natural service may serve up to 100 cows per year and an AI bull may sire up to 50 000 calves per year. The selection of suitable bulls to pass on their genes to future generations is thus of paramount importance. However, the correct choice of cows from which to produce calves can also have an impact. Techniques such as MOET (multiple ovulation and embryo transfer) increase the number of offspring that a cow can produce and increase the importance of effective methods of selecting appropriate females. They can therefore increase the rate of genetic progress, although probably not to the same extent as by the use of AI. Similarly, other novel techniques such as the splitting and cloning of embryos, also described in Chapter 13, may increase the speed at which genetic improvements can be made. Effective selection of the female is also of importance when choosing cows that are to be the mothers of potential future AI sires.

Selection priorities will depend on whether the cow is predominantly a dual-purpose animal, as in most of mainland Europe and some developing countries, or specifically developed for either milk or meat, as in areas such as North America and Australasia. In the UK, cattle production falls between these two extremes, although there has been a trend towards specialist milk-producing cows, notably the Holstein, over the last few decades. The UK is also unusual in that the majority of home-produced beef is a by-product of the dairy herd (see Chapter 1). This can lead to problems in terms of selection of appropriate sires for breeding with dairy cows.

Genetic inheritance

The characteristics exhibited by an animal – its phenotype – e.g., milk yield and growth rate, are dependent on two factors:

(1) the genes that it inherits from its parents, i.e., its genotype
(2) the effects of the environment in which the animal is kept.

These two factors are commonly referred to as 'nature' and 'nurture', particularly in the human context.

A particular characteristic or phenotype may be qualitative or quantitative. Qualitative traits are absolute, e.g., coat colour, and are usually controlled by one or a few genes. Polledness in the Aberdeen Angus breed is an example of a character determined by a single gene. Quantitative characteristics, such as milk yield and growth rate, are widely variable, and these tend to be controlled by a larger number of additive genes. Thousands of different genes control milk production, affecting a large variety of factors which together influence production. These factors include food intake, metabolic efficiency and the partition of nutrients between mammary and other needs.

The objective of the cattle breeder is to produce animals that have inherited, from their parents, combinations of genes that influence production and conformation traits in a desirable way. In general, the breeder aims to produce animals of equal or improved performance to that of the parents. The science of applied genetics is highly dependent on statistical probabilities. This usually means that the use of genetically superior sires and dams is more likely to produce superior progeny than the use of inferior ones. Selection is the process of choosing which animals are genetically superior so that these can be used for breeding. Selection methods are used to provide an estimate of the breeding value (BV) of the potential parent.

It will be recalled from Chapter 5 that fertilization is the process by which the maternal and paternal pronuclei, each containing the haploid number of chromosomes (30), fuse to form the zygote containing the diploid number (60) of chromosomes. Thus the embryonic calf receives chromosomes, the genetic material, from each of its parents. Each chromosome contains a large number of genes, each of which is a strand of DNA comprising a specific sequence of the four bases, adenine, guanine, cytosine and thymine. The sequence of these bases in the gene determines the primary structure of proteins synthesized in the cell.

Heritability

Some of the more important traits for beef and milk production are shown in Table 15.1. Heritability expressed in percentage terms, is a measure of the degree to which a particular trait can be influenced by genetics. The higher the heritability of a trait the easier it is to improve that trait by genetic selection. For example, the heritability of milk yield is regarded as moderate, whereas those of beefing traits are relatively high.

Selection may be carried out on a 'tandem' involving the progressive improvement of a single trait to a certain end point, after which another single trait is chosen for selection and improvement. Alternatively there could be simultaneous selection for a combination of traits, using a selection index. This is a score of overall genetic merit of the animals available for selection, based on their own or their relatives' performance in the traits of interest. The traits

Table 15.1 Heritability estimates of some important traits in cattle.

Trait	Heritability (%)	Reference
Dairy		
Milk yield	25–35	a
Total solids	25–30	a
Fat yield	25–35	a
Protein yield	25–30	a
Lactose and minerals	25–32	a
Solids not fat yield	25–30	a
Fat percentage	50–60	a
Protein percentage	45–55	a
Total solids percentage	50–65	a
Solids not fat percentage	55–65	a
Fore udder attachment	20, 29	b, c
Udder support	16	b, c
Udder depth	29, 33	b, c
Beef		
Birth weight	40	d
Weaning weight	30	d
Yearling weight	50	d
Feed conversion efficiency	40	d
Conformation	40	d
Carcase fat cover	50	d
Saleable meat yield percentage	40	d

[a] ADAS (1982).
[b] MMB (1986).
[c] Meyer *et al.* (1987).
[d] Allen & Kilkenny (1984).

are differentially weighted to take account of their relative importance. Indices are constantly being improved, incorporating, for example, a financial element and including traits such as longevity. For full details of such indices see Simm (1998). In general, as the number of traits selected at any one time increases, so the heritability of each is decreased.

Specific objectives in dairy cattle selection

These include:

(1) the increase in milk yield and its compositional quality
(2) the improvement of conformation including udder and feet
(3) the improvement of beef merit
(4) the improvement of fertility.

Milk yield, milk quality and conformation can all be improved by genetic means, as can beef merit. However, improvement of beef merit is often achieved at the expense of improvement in milk traits. Therefore in the past the improvement of beef merit has been a low-priority objective in the dairy herd and this is exemplified by the increasing Holstein influence (an extreme dairy type) in the British dairy herd. Beef merit can be important in choosing a terminal sire that will produce a calf to be reared for beef, but not produce any offspring itself. Such a bull may be used in Holstein cows that are not selected to produce replacements for the dairy herd.

Unfortunately, fertility has a low heritability and it is greatly affected by the environment. Therefore it is difficult to improve fertility by selection. However, there is a body of opinion that believes that an increase in milk yield over the last five decades or so has brought about a decrease in dairy herd fertility. As was seen in Chapter 1, there is a negative association between the two, but the degree to which genetics and management have contributed to this is debatable. Pryce *et al.* (2002) showed that selecting for milk yield alone would result in an increase of 768 kg of milk for every standard deviation change in the index, but that this would be accompanied by an increase of 4.46 days in the calving interval and a reduction of 0.41 body condition score units. The link between low condition score and impaired fertility has already been highlighted. There is thus a risk of *reducing* fertility by inappropriate selection. It must also be remembered that specific aspects of fertility, such as a propensity to cystic ovarian disease or detectable embryo/fetal loss, may be more heritable than overall indices, such as calving interval, which are controlled by a huge number of genes and which are highly sensitive to environmental and management effects.

In beef cattle, bull selection is made on the basis of weight gain or high weight for age. The advantages are that these parameters are simple to measure, their heritability is high and faster growth is associated with efficient feed conversion and with lean growth, these two also being desirable traits. However, rate of gain is also correlated to liveweight at birth and therefore selection for very high growth rates can lead to problems of dystocia.

Methods of testing for selection of sires

There is a greater selection intensity for sires than for dams, i.e., selected animals are likely to be of greater genetic merit since the number of sires required is much smaller than the number of dams. This is particularly true due to the extensive use of AI. Therefore sires can be tested far more rigorously than dams.

A variety of testing methods for the identification of genetically superior animals are available. These include performance testing, lifetime performance recording, pedigree records, progeny testing, sib performance and various combinations of these. Progeny testing is widely used in the UK and in many parts of the world and therefore merits discussion in some detail.

The progeny test

Obviously, a bull cannot be evaluated directly for the traits of most interest, such as milk yield and composition. This is overcome by evaluating the performance of a large number of his offspring in progeny testing. This is probably the most accurate selection test since it directly assesses the traits of interest in the test sire's progeny, evaluating the bull's ability to pass on desirable characteristics. The evaluation of large numbers of animals adds to the accuracy of this form of testing. However, it is very expensive and time consuming; the generation interval (i.e., the time between birth of the potential sire and its general usage as a sire) may be five or more years. Consequently, only a limited number of bulls are progeny tested.

Progeny testing of dairy bulls involves the mating of the bull under test to a number of cows in several herds using AI and recording the performance of the daughters in their first lactation. The performance of the daughters is compared with that of contemporary heifers that are daughters of other bulls. This so-called contemporary comparison is thus an estimate of the difference in the performance of a bull's daughters from that of contemporaries. A valid contemporary comparison requires that:

- a representative number of cows are in the test
- there is no bias in selection of cows used
- cows in a herd are managed in a similar way
- factors such as age, month of calving and weight and body condition at calving can all be corrected for.

In recent years the improved contemporary comparison (ICC) has been introduced which overcomes some of the problems of bias that had been associated with the contemporary comparison. The procedure used in the UK is similar to that used in other countries with highly developed dairy industries, e.g., the USA, Canada and New Zealand. It relies on the use of a best linear unbiased prediction (BLUP), which takes account of the overall genetic trend during the progeny test and the effects of using different contemporaries for comparison in different herds. A large, fixed, genetic database (approximately 24000 bulls) is used for comparison using the ICC and adjustments are made for month of calving, age at first calving and differences in merit between sires of the contemporaries. Progeny testing of dairy bulls is carried out in the UK by the AI organizations and ICCs are given for weight of milk, fat and protein and percentage fat and protein.

Most major AI companies worldwide use progeny testing to evaluate dairy bulls. Relatively little progeny testing of beef bulls is carried out in the UK. Genus operates a scheme that assesses the progeny of beef bulls and dairy cows. The progeny (25 per bull) of certain bulls are collected and reared on a central station on a standard semi-intensive beef production system and their performance is monitored. The measurements taken include liveweight gain and carcass characteristics including weight, fatness and shape. The test also allows some assessment of potential calving difficulties.

Sire fertility

In addition to evaluation of potential AI sires for their ability to impart superior characteristics to their offspring, an evaluation should be made of their own fertility. Not enough attention has been paid to this in the past, but there is considerable variation between the conception rates achieved by different bulls. Anzar *et al.* (2002), using flow cytometry, were able to measure significant differences in the percentage of apoptotic (degenerating) sperm among bulls and suggested that this could be one of the reasons for poor fertility in breeding bulls. A combination of non-return rate data obtained from tested progeny, semen tests such as those of Anzar *et al.* (2002) and results from in vitro fertilization (see, for example, Ward *et al.*, 2003) could possibly be used to evaluate a bull's fertility before his semen goes on sale.

Methods of testing for selection of dams

Dairy cows

There are a number of aids to decision making in terms of selection of cows for breeding. These can give guidance to the producer as to whether cows should be put to a nominated bull, bull of the day, a beef bull, or culled. The essential items that the milk producer is interested in are milk yield, fat and protein, since he is currently paid a bonus on the compositional quality. Good records should also be kept of all aspects of fertility, including the number of services required for conception in each lactation, and the incidence of particular problems such as cystic ovarian disease.

A simple guide to cow selection is the construction of a cow production index (CPI) (see ADAS, 1982) in which cows within a herd are ranked on the basis of their 'solids' yield in their most recent lactation, corrected for the lactation number. Attempts to improve CPIs have emphasized a need to include fertility parameters. Royal *et al.* (2002), using milk progesterone profile data, estimated the heritability for interval to commencement of luteal activity postpartum, length of the first luteal phase and occurrence of one type of persistent corpus luteum as 0.16, 0.17 and 0.13, respectively, as compared to <0.05 for traditional measurements of fertility such as calving interval, days open and non-return rate.

Other traits that may be selected for in a production index include conformation, udder conformation and resistance to mastitis.

Summary

Most genetic progress is likely to be made through the selection of bulls, since each individual is capable of producing a relatively large number of offspring. However, the choice of cows used to breed replacements is also important, not least because some specific fertility disorders, as well as production and conformation characteristics, can be relatively highly heritable. Techniques such as MOET increase the contribution from female stock.

The basic principles of parent selection have been covered in this chapter, but the subject is large and complex and for further information the reader is referred to a number of specialist publications listed in the References. Particular attention is drawn to Simm (1998), not least for a detailed account of selection indices.

References

ADAS (1982) *An Introduction to Cattle Breeding*, No. 3, Booket 2405.

Allen, D.M. & Kilkenny, J.B. (1984) *Planned Beef Production*, 2nd edn. Blackwell Science, Oxford.

Anzar, M., He, L., Buhr, M.M., Kroetsch, T.G. & Pauls, K.P. (2002) *Biology of Reproduction*, **66**, 354–360.

Meyer, K., Brotherstone, S. & Hill, W.G. (1987) *Animal Production*, **44**, 1.

MMB (1986) *Report of the Breeding and Production Organisation*, **33**, 50.

Pryce, J.E., Coffey, M.P., Brotherstone, S.H. & Woolliams, J.A. (2002) *Journal of Dairy Science*, **85**, 1590–1595.

Royal, M.D., Flint, A.P. & Woolliams, J.A. (2002) *Journal of Dairy Science*, **85**, 958–967.

Simm, G. (1998) *Genetic Improvement of Cattle and Sheep*. Farming Press, Ipswich.

Ward, F., Rizos, D., Boland, M.P. & Lonergan, P. (2003) *Theriogenology*, **59**, 1575–1584.

Index

abortion 148, 186–8
accessory organs (*see* male sex organs)
acrosome 31
acrosome reaction 56, 57
adenohypophysis (*see* pituitary, anterior)
adhesions 174–5
adrenal 33, 75, 76
adrenal cortex 33
adrenocorticotrophic hormone (ACTH) 16
ageing
  cows 183–4
  ova 183
aldosterone 33
allantois 60–61
alveolus 74
amnion 60
amniotic sac 61
ampulla 23, 56
androgenized steers 105
antibiotics 132, 160, 161
artificial insemination (AI) 28, 124–39
  advantages 124–6
  cost effectiveness 125
  in developing countries 127
  disease control 125
  do-it-yourself (DIY) 127, 133
  during pregnancy 182–3
  fixed time 107, 136, 145
  flexibility 126
  genetic gain 126
  'gun' 137–8
  history of 126–7
  safety 125
  technique 134–8
  timing 134–6
artificial vagina 28, 128

balanoposthitis 156
ballotement (*see* pregnancy, diagnosis)
best linear unbiased prediction (BLUP) 235
betamethasone (*see* corticosteroids)

blastocyst 58
block calving 4
body condition 85, 224–6
bovine herpes virus 163
bovine leucocyte (BLAD) 157
bovine spongiform encephalitis (BSE) 2
bovine trophoblast protein (*see* pregnancy-specific proteins)
bovine viral diarrhoea 163
bovine pregnancy associated glycoprotein (BPAG) (*see* pregnancy-specific proteins)
breeding policy 222–3
breeding value 232
Brucella abortus 162–3
bulbo-cavernosus muscles 37
bulbo-urethral glands 16, 20
bulling 95

calf
  rearing 216–18
  weight 207
calving
  autumn 4
  spring 4
  summer 4
calving interval 8
calving patterns 3, 220–21
calving rate 7
calving season 6
calving to conception interval 8
Campylobacter fetus 161
capacitation 56–7
caruncles 22, 61
cerebral cortex 13
cervix 13, 21
chamise sanitaire 137, 138, 162
chimerism 157
cholesterol 27
CIDRb (*see* controlled internal drug releaser, bovine)
cleavage 58
clenbuterol 74

238

9 781405 115452